Exercise-Induced Bronchoconstriction

Editor

SANDRA D. ANDERSON

IMMUNOLOGY AND ALLERGY CLINICS OF NORTH AMERICA

www.immunology.theclinics.com

Consulting Editor
RAFEUL ALAM

August 2013 • Volume 33 • Number 3

ELSEVIER

1600 John F. Kennedy Boulevard • Suite 1800 • Philadelphia, Pennsylvania, 19103-2899

http://www.theclinics.com

IMMUNOLOGY AND ALLERGY CLINICS OF NORTH AMERICA Volume 33, Number 3

August 2013 ISSN 0889-8561, ISBN-13: 978-0-323-18607-0

Editor: Pamela Hetherington

Immunology and Allergy Clinics of North America (ISSN 0889-8561) is published quarterly by Elsevier Inc., 360 Park Avenue South, New York, NY 10010-1710. Months of issue are February, May, August, and November. Periodicals postage paid at New York, NY and additional mailing offices. Subscription prices are $306.00 per year for US individuals, $442.00 per year for US institutions, $144.00 per year for US students and residents, $375.00 per year for Canadian individuals, $209.00 per year for Canadian students, $547.00 per year for Canadian institutions, $425.00 per year for international individuals, $547.00 per year for international institutions, $209.00 per year for international students. To receive student/resident rate, orders must be accompanied by name of affiliated institution, date of term, and the *signature* of program/residency coordinator on institution letterhead. Orders will be billed at individual rate until proof of status is received. Foreign air speed delivery is included in all *Clinics* subscription prices. All prices are subject to change without notice. **POSTMASTER:** Send address changes to *Immunology and Allergy Clinics of North America,* Elsevier Health Sciences Division, Subscription Customer Service, 3251 Riverport Lane, Maryland Heights, MO 63043. **Customer Service: 1-800-654-2452 (U.S. and Canada); 314-447-8871 (outside U.S. and Canada). Fax: 314-447-8029. E-mail: journalscustomerservice-usa@elsevier.com (for print support); journalsonlinesupport-usa@elsevier.com (for online support).**

Reprints. For copies of 100 or more, of articles in this publication, please contact the Commercial Reprints Department, Elsevier Inc., 360 Park Avenue South, New York, New York 10010-1710. Tel. (212) 633-3812, Fax: (212) 462-1935, E-mail: reprints@elsevier.com.

Immunology and Allergy Clinics of North America is covered in MEDLINE/PubMed (Index Medicus), Current Contents/Life Sciences, Science Citation Index, ISI/BIOMED, Chemical Abstracts, and EMBASE/Excerpta Medica.

Printed and bound by CPI Group (UK) Ltd, Croydon, CR0 4YY
Transferred to digital print 2013

Contributors

CONSULTING EDITOR

RAFEUL ALAM, MD, PhD
Professor and Chief, Division of Allergy and Immunology, National Jewish Health, University of Colorado Denver School of Medicine, Denver, Colorado

EDITOR

SANDRA D. ANDERSON, PhD, DSC, MD(HON)
Clinical Professor, Department of Respiratory and Sleep Medicine, Royal Prince Alfred Hospital, Camperdown, New South Wales, Australia

AUTHORS

MOIRA L. AITKEN, MD
Division of Pulmonary and Critical Care, Department of Medicine, University of Washington, Seattle, Washington

WILLIAM A. ALTEMEIER, MD
Division of Pulmonary and Critical Care, Department of Medicine, University of Washington, Seattle, Washington

SANDRA D. ANDERSON, PhD, DSc, MD(Hon)
Clinical Professor, Department of Respiratory and Sleep Medicine, Royal Prince Alfred Hospital, Camperdown, New South Wales, Australia

VIBEKE BACKER, MD, DMSci
Professor, Respiratory Research Unit, Department of Respiratory Medicine, Bispebjerg Hospital, University of Copenhagen, Copenhagen NV, Denmark

VALÉRIE BOUGAULT, PhD
Associate Professor, Faculty of Sport Sciences, Université Lille Nord de France (Lille 2 University of Health and Law), Lille, France

LOUIS-PHILIPPE BOULET, MD, FCCP
Pneumologist, Institut Universitaire de Cardiologie et de Pneumologie, Québec City, Québec, Canada

JOHN D. BRANNAN, PhD
Hospital Scientist, Department of Respiratory and Sleep Medicine, Westmead Hospital, University of Sydney, Westmead, New South Wales, Australia

BARBRO DAHLÉN, MD, PhD
Lung and Allergy Research, Division of Respiratory Medicine and Allergy, Department of Medicine, Karolinska University Hospital Huddinge; Centre for Allergy Research, Karolinska Institutet, Stockholm, Sweden

SVEN-ERIK DAHLÉN, MD, PhD
Division of Physiology, The National Institute of Environmental Medicine; Centre for Allergy Research, Karolinska Institutet, Stockholm, Sweden

JEAN M.M. DRIESSEN, MD, PhD
Specialist in Training, Department of Pediatrics, Medisch Spectrum Twente, Enschede; Department of Sports Medicine, Tjongerschans Hospital, Heerenveen, The Netherlands

KENNETH D. FITCH, MD, MBBS, DSc (Hon), FACRM, FACSP
Adjunct Professor, School of Sports Science, Exercise and Health, University of Western Australia, Crawley, Western Australia, Australia

SIMON GODFREY, MD, PhD, FRCP, FRCPCH
Emeritus Professor of Pediatrics, Hadassah Hebrew University, Jerusalem, Israel

TEAL S. HALLSTRAND, MD, MPH
Division of Pulmonary and Critical Care, Department of Medicine, Associate Professor of Medicine, University of Washington, Seattle, Washington

WILLIAM R. HENDERSON Jr, MD
Division of Allergy and Infectious Diseases, Department of Medicine, University of Washington, Seattle, Washington

ELIN T.G. KERSTEN, MD
Department of Pediatrics, Medisch Spectrum Twente, Enschede; Department of Pediatric Pulmonology, GRIAC Research Institute, Beatrix Children's Hospital, University Medical Center Groningen, Groningen, The Netherlands

PASCALE KIPPELEN, PhD
Senior Lecturer, Centre for Sports Medicine and Human Performance, Brunel University, Uxbridge, Middlesex, United Kingdom

JOHAN LARSSON, MD
PhD Student, Lung and Allergy Research, Division of Respiratory Medicine and Allergy, Department of Medicine, Karolinska University Hospital Huddinge; Division of Physiology, The National Institute of Environmental Medicine; Centre for Allergy Research, Karolinska Institutet, Stockholm, Sweden

CELESTE PORSBJERG, MD, PhD
Staff Respiratory Specialist, Respiratory Research Unit, Department of Respiratory Medicine, Bispebjerg Hospital, University of Copenhagen, Copenhagen NV, Denmark

KENNETH W. RUNDELL, PhD
Medical Affairs Consultant, Pharmaxis Inc, Philadelphia; Professor of Basic Sciences, Commonwealth Medical College, Scranton, Pennsylvania

MALCOLM SUE-CHU, MB ChB, PhD
Consultant Pulmonologist, Department of Thoracic Medicine, Trondheim University Hospital, St Olavs Hospital; Associate Professor, Institute of Circulation and Imaging, Norwegian University of Science and Technology, Trondheim, Norway

ASGER SVERRILD, MD
PhD Student, Respiratory Research Unit, Department of Respiratory Medicine, Bispebjerg Hospital, University of Copenhagen, Copenhagen NV, Denmark

BERNARD J. THIO, MD, PhD
Department of Pediatrics, Medisch Spectrum Twente, Enschede, The Netherlands

JANNEKE C. VAN LEEUWEN, MD
Specialist in Training, Department of Pediatrics, Medisch Spectrum Twente, Enschede; Department of Pediatric Pulmonology, GRIAC Research Institute, Beatrix Children's Hospital, University Medical Center Groningen, Groningen, The Netherlands

Contents

> This article examines in detail the history of more than half a century of investigations into elucidating the causation of exercise-induced bronchoconstriction. Despite earnest attempts by many researchers from many countries, answers to some pivotal questions await the next generation of investigators into exercise-induced bronchoconstriction.

> This article presents the various potential mechanisms responsible for the development of exercise-induced bronchoconstriction (EIB). Although the etiology of EIB is multifactorial, and the physiologic processes involved may vary between individuals (especially between those with and without asthma), drying of the small airways with an associated inflammatory response seems prerequisite for EIB. Dysregulated repair processes following exercise-induced airway epithelial injury may also serve as basis for EIB development/progression.

> A susceptible group of subjects with asthma develops airflow obstruction in response to the transfer of water out of the airways during exercise. The transfer of water or the challenge with a hypertonic solution serves as a strong stimulus to the airway epithelium. Susceptible subjects have epithelial shedding into the airway lumen, and airway inflammation that leads to the overproduction of leukotrienes and other eicosanoids following exercise challenge. The sensory nerves of the airways may serve as a critical link that mediates the effect of eicosanoids, leading to bronchoconstriction and mucus production in response to exercise challenge.

This article discusses the available literature on refractoriness in exercise-induced bronchoconstriction, namely, a decrease in airway responsiveness with repeated exercise challenges. The mechanisms of this naturally occurring protective feature is unknown. Reviewing previous studies together with findings in more recent studies, the authors propose desensitization of the G protein–coupled cysteinyl leukotriene receptor$_1$ as the mechanism of refractoriness and that this desensitization occurs as a result of interplay between leukotrienes and prostaglandins.

Exercise-induced bronchoconstriction (EIB) describes the transient narrowing of the airways during, and particularly after exercise and occurs commonly in asthmatic individuals. Limitation of exercise capacity is a frequent complaint in all age groups, and severity of EIB ranges from mild impairment of performance to severe bronchospasm and a large reduction in FEV_1. Treatment of EIB varies from daily to less frequent therapy, depending on the level of activity. In this article, the authors evaluate the treatment possibilities before, during, and after exercise. They also review medications currently used to treat EIB.

Respiratory symptoms and asthma control questionnaires are poor predictors of the presence or severity of exercise-induced bronchoconstriction (EIB), and objective measurement is recommended. To optimize the chance of a positive test result, there are several factors to consider when exercising patients for EIB, including the ventilation achieved and sustained during exercise, water content of the inspired air, and the natural variability of the response. The high rate of negative exercise test results has led to the development of surrogates to identify EIB in laboratory or office settings, including eucapnic voluntary hyperpnea of dry air and inhalation of hyperosmolar aerosols.

Recent research shows important differences in exercise-induced bronchoconstriction (EIB) between children and adults, suggesting a different pathophysiology of EIB in children. Although exercise can trigger classic symptoms of asthma, in children symptoms can be subtle and nonspecific; parents, children, and clinicians often do not recognize EIB. With an age-adjusted protocol, an exercise challenge test can be performed in children as young as 3 years of age. However, an alternative challenge test is sometimes necessary to assess potential for EIB in children. This review summarizes age-related features of EIB and recommendations for assessing EIB in young children and adolescents.

Concerns have been expressed about the possible detrimental effects of chlorine derivatives in indoor swimming pool environments. Indeed, a controversy has arisen regarding the possibility that chlorine commonly used worldwide as a disinfectant favors the development of asthma and allergic diseases. The effects of swimming in indoor chlorinated pools on the airways in recreational and elite swimmers are presented. Recent studies on the influence of swimming on airway inflammation and remodeling in competitive swimmers, and the phenotypic characteristics of asthma in this population are reviewed. Preventative measures that could potentially reduce the untoward effects of pool environment on airways of swimmers are discussed.

A higher prevalence of airway hyperresponsiveness, airway remodeling, and asthma has been identified among athletes who compete and train in environmental conditions of cold dry air and/or high air pollution. Repeated long-duration exposure to cold/dry air at high minute ventilation rates can cause airway damage. Competition or training at venues close to busy roadways, or in indoor ice arenas or chlorinated swimming pools, harbors a risk for acute and chronic airway disorders from high pollutant exposure. This article discusses the effects of these harsh environments on the airways, and summarizes potential mechanisms and prevalence of airway disorders in elite athletes.

The role of epithelial injury is an unanswered question in those with established asthma and in elite athletes who develop features of asthma and exercise-induced bronchorestriction (EIB) after years of training. The movement of water in response to changes in osmolarity is likely to be an important signal to the epithelium that may be central to the onset of EIB. It is generally accepted that the mast cell and its mediators play a major role in EIB and the presence of eosinophils is likely to enhance EIB severity.

IMMUNOLOGY AND ALLERGY CLINICS OF NORTH AMERICA

Erratum

With regard to the article "Rhinosinusitis and Nasal Polyps in Aspirin-Exacerbated Respiratory Disease," by Joaquim Mullol, MD, PhD and César Picado, MD, PhD, which appeared in *Immunology and Allergy Clinics of North America,* May 2013 33(2):163-176, the publisher would like to clarify that Table 1 on page 171 and Table 2 on page 172 have incorrect credit lines. The correct credit line for both tables is: Fokkens WJ, Lund V, Mullol J, et al. EPOS 2012: European position paper on rhinosinusitis and nasal polyps 2012. Rhinology 2012;50 (Suppl 23):1–298.

Foreword

Exercise, Our Breathing, and Our Health

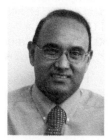

Rafeul Alam, MD, PhD
Consulting Editor

Exercise is a form of physical stress that elicits a variety of biological responses. Most of these responses have a positive effect on our body and mind. For this reason, we actively promote exercise to our patients. Unfortunately, many patients are unable to tolerate exercise. They experience symptoms of asthma, urticaria, angioedema, and even life-threatening anaphylaxis. How physical exercise induces bronchospasm and other mast cell activation-related syndromes has been the subject of active research for many years. Bronchospasm in a susceptible asthmatic patient occurs not only in response to exercise but also to a sudden change in weather or barometric pressure. How these diverse forms of physical stress elicit a cellular response that results in asthma exacerbation remains a fascinating subject. The current consensus opinion on pathogenesis of exercise-induced asthma relies on changes in osmolality and ionic tonicity of the extracellular fluid. Neuronal and nonneuronal cells in the airways express a variety of osmoreceptors and ion channels that respond to the changes in osmolality and ionic strength. How activation of these osmoreceptors and ion channels leads to activation of mast cells and inflammatory and airway cells need further investigation. Many ion channels regulate intracellular calcium homeostasis, which is important for mast cell activation. Mast cells express a variety of calcium ion channels (Orai 1, 2, and 3, L-type voltage-gated calcium channels), calcium and other cation channels (P2X, transient receptor potential—TRP channels), potassium, and chloride channels.[1,2] Exercise alters body heat and induces transient acidosis, both of which activate TRPV1 (TRP vanilloid 1) channel. Reactive oxygen species and kinins generated during exercise activate the TRPA1 (TRP ankyrin 1) channel. Both TRPV1 and TRPA1 are expressed on mast cells. It would be important to know if exercise alters the function of these ion channels on mast cells and if their blockade prevents exercise-induced asthma.

Supported by NIH Grants RO1 AI091614, PPG HL 36577, and N01 HHSN272200700048C.

Immunol Allergy Clin N Am 33 (2013) xiii–xiv
http://dx.doi.org/10.1016/j.iac.2013.05.002
0889-8561/13/$ – see front matter © 2013 Published by Elsevier Inc.

immunology.theclinics.com

To update us on this important topic, I have invited Dr Sandra Anderson, a leader and an accomplished scientist in the field, to lead this issue. She has brought together an outstanding group of scientists and clinical investigators, who present the state of the art in the field.

Rafeul Alam, MD, PhD
Division of Allergy and Immunology
National Jewish Health
University of Colorado Denver
1400 Jackson Street
Denver, CO 80206, USA

E-mail address:
alamr@njhealth.org

REFERENCES

1. Ashmole I, Bradding P. Ion channels regulating mast cell biology. ClinExp Allergy 2013;43:491–502.
2. Smith PK, Nilius B. Transient receptor potentials (TRPs) and anaphylaxis. Curr Allergy Asthma Rep 2013;13:93–100.

Preface

Exercise-Induced bronchoconstriction

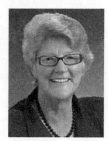

Sandra D. Anderson, PhD, DSc, MD(Hon)
Editor

The invitation by the editor, Rafeul Alam, to guest edit this issue on exercise-induced bronchoconstriction (EIB) allowed me to bring together investigators from physiology to cellular biology of EIB. The preface contains information on how some of the contributors came together and identifies some conferences that helped broaden the scientific research in EIB in asthmatic children to include healthy elite athletes. The contributors come from Australia, Canada, Denmark, England, France, Israel, Sweden, Netherlands, and the United States and trained in pediatric, respiratory, and sports medicine and science. Most have either obtained a doctoral degree in EIB or supervised one.

My first encounter with EIB was at Royal Prince Alfred Hospital, in Sydney, in 1968. In January 1970 I started research in EIB with Simon Godfrey in the Department of Paediatrics at the Brompton Hospital in London. Over the next 3 years, under Simon's enthusiastic guidance, a group of us carried out many studies on various aspects of EIB.

In 1968 Ken Fitch from Perth, Australia observed severe EIB when supervising an exercise test on an 18-year-old asthmatic Olympic swimmer, who 3 months later won an Olympic Gold Medal in Mexico. This induced Ken to do his MD in EIB. Both Simon and Ken's laboratories were coincidentally investigating the effect of different forms of exercise to provoke EIB. In 1971, both laboratories reported running as the most provocative exercise. Being ahead of their time, Ken and Simon wrote an article in 1976 on the topic of Asthma and Athletic Performance. They now celebrate the 50 years of research since the modern description of EIB in children by R.S. Jones of Liverpool, United Kingdom, in 1962. In 1973 Simon moved to the Hammersmith Hospital and later, in 1977, to Israel, where he continued his studies, among many others, on refractoriness and EIB. The article by Larsson and coworkers discusses these early studies and presents a new hypothesis to explain refractoriness following EIB.

Immunol Allergy Clin N Am 33 (2013) xv–xvii
http://dx.doi.org/10.1016/j.iac.2013.05.001
0889-8561/13/$ – see front matter © 2013 Published by Elsevier Inc.
immunology.theclinics.com

On my return to Sydney we studied the effects of β_2-agonists and in 1975-1976 reported that tablets failed to inhibit EIB, relative to an inhaled aerosol, when both gave an equivalent bronchodilator effect. The mast cell, situated superficially in the airway, was proposed as a second site of action for the inhaled β_2-agonist to prevent EIB. Down-regulation of mast cell β_2-receptors is now recognized as a contributing factor to the tolerance that develops to β_2-agonists. Vibeke Backer writes about the benefits and limitations of β_2-agonists and other drugs in the treatment of EIB.

In May 1982 a symposium was held in Oslo, Norway (The Asthmatic Child in Sport and Play. Oseid S, Edwards A, editors. Bath, UK: Pitman Press: 1983:1–396). Most topics related to EIB and included standardization of testing, the effect of climatic conditions, the role of mast cell mediators, refractoriness, and the effect of both short and prolonged periods of exercise. This meeting reflected the growing interest in EIB research by 1982.

In 1984 a conference was held in Palm Springs on Special Problems and Management of Allergic Athletes (J Allergy Clin Immunol 1984;73(5 Part 2):629–748). In addition to the assessment and treatment of EIB, the topics included doping, air pollution, and the management of allergic Olympic athletes. The osmotic hypothesis, as an alternative to the cooling hypothesis, of EIB was presented for the first time. In part, this hypothesis was based on the finding, by the Perth and Sydney groups, that severe EIB occurred when hot dry air was inhaled during exercise. Later, in 1984, at the American Thoracic Society (ATS) in Miami, Moira Aitkin from Seattle reporting similar findings with hot dry air.

The osmotic hypothesis was the first of a series of articles on calculating water loss from the airway surface by E. Daviskas. The concepts of water loss from the airway surface ultimately led to the proposal that airway injury from water loss may be important in the pathogenesis of EIB, particularly in athletes. The topic is covered by Pascale Kippelen and me in the second article. One of the aspects of water loss and airway injury is the shedding of the airway epithelium, a subject studied by Teal Hallstrand. Since his presentation at ATS in 1996, Teal has taken the subject of EIB from the physiologic aspects to molecular biology. His article on cells and mediators in EIB demonstrates how sophisticated EIB research is today.

In 1997 at a conference in Oslo, Norway (Exercise-induced Asthma and Sports in Asthma. Carlsen KH, Ibsen TB, editors. Copenhagen: Munksgaard; 1999:1–114), Malcolm Sue Chu and colleagues reported pathologic and inflammatory changes in the airways of healthy elite cross-country skiers. A few years later in 1999, Ken Rundell, a sports physiologist, also studying cold weather athletes at the US Olympic Committee facility at Lake Placid, New York, attended an International Olympic Committee conference held in Sydney. In 2001 he reported that the respiratory symptoms, associated with exercise and asthma, were neither sensitive nor specific for predicting EIB. This study confirmed the need for objective tests for a correct diagnosis to be made. A later study reported eucapnic voluntary hyperpnea (EVH) to be a reliable test to identify EIB in elite cold-weather athletes. Ken and Malcolm write on air quality and EIB.

In 2003, Pascale Kippelen, also a sports physiologist, came from Montpellier in France to do a post-doctoral in Sydney. At the time our laboratory was active in assessing defense force recruits and intending scuba divers for asthma and EIB. It was the need to assess "healthy" subjects for EIB and the low yield for exercise to identify EIB that had led John Brannan and me to use surrogates such as EVH and mannitol to identify potential for EIB. Exercise and these surrogates for exercise are discussed in the article on assessment of EIB. At that time, we were working on the urinary excretion of mediators following inhalation of mannitol with Sven Erik and Barbro Dahlen from the Karolinska Institute in Stockholm, who had published on mediators in EIB some years earlier. With Pascale, the studies were extended to include mediators following EVH. Johan Larsson joined the Dahlens for his PhD and remains involved with studies with Pascale, who is now in London.

In 2001 Ken Fitch involved me in a meeting at the IOC headquarters in Lausanne to discuss testing for asthma. The outcome was a policy requiring athletes, seeking to use a β_2-agonist before an event, to submit the results of provocation tests before the Winter and Summer Olympics of 2002 and 2004. Over the years, Ken Fitch met Ken Rundell, Pascale Kippelen, Malcolm Sue Chu, Louis-Philippe Boulet, Vibeke Backer, and Valerie Bougault and most came together at a second meeting in Lausanne in 2008. Valerie and Louis-Philippe were studying the swimming pool environment and athletes. Their findings were timely, as swimmers represented a high proportion of the athletes taking β_2-agonists. They write here on airway disorders and the swimming pool.

At the Winter Games in Vancouver (2006) and the Summer Games in Beijing (2008), Fitch noted that most ($\sim 62\%$) athletes reporting asthma for the first time were over the age of 23 years. Malcolm's study in young skiers, showing a high percentage with hyperresponsiveness to methacholine, supported both the earlier and the later findings of Louis-Philippe's group in cold weather athletes and swimmers. All these observations suggest that years of training, as well as the environment, may be important in the pathogenesis of hyperresponsive airways and EIB and emphasize the need to have strategies to prevent airway injury. Ken Fitch is to be commended for all his effort, through his long membership of the IOC Medical Commission, to encourage testing and measurement in athletes and to monitor use of β_2-agonists. This approach has resulted in better recognition and treatment of asthma in athletes, an outcome in keeping with a focus on the health of athletes. In 2011 the responsibility for approval of drugs was taken over by the World Anti-Doping Authority and testing is now no longer required to use the commonly available aerosols of β_2-agonists. In 2011 in Monaco at an IOC Conference, many writing here presented at a symposium entitled Intensive Exercise and Respiratory Health (Br J Sports Med 2012;46(6):379-421; Br J Sports Med 2012;46(7):471-476).

Boony Thio, a pediatrician from The Netherlands, came to Sydney for 3 months in December 2008 and we discussed tolerance to β_2-agonists and EIB. A few years later, I met Boony's PhD students, Elin Kersten, Jean Driessen, and Janneke Van Leeuwen. They reported, in a pilot study, the benefit of withdrawing β_2-agonists on EIB severity. They were using a new skating rink for testing for EIB. The children ran on a treadmill in environmental conditions similar to those outside. They demonstrated breakthrough EIB during exercise in a large proportion of asthmatic children. They also developed a new test for EIB in very young children using a jumping castle. They write on the assessment of EIB in adolescents and young children. EIB research seems to be returning to where it started...enthusiastic pediatricians like R.S. Jones and Simon Godfrey guiding students in the study of EIB in children. In the last article, this group and other members of the younger generation ask where to from here for EIB and what are the unanswered questions.

Finally, I would like to thank all the contributors for their enthusiasm in writing for this issue and for being on time with both their original and revised articles.

Sandra D. Anderson, PhD, DSc, MD(Hon)
Department of Respiratory and Sleep Medicine
Royal Prince Alfred Hospital
Camperdown, New South Wales 2050, Australia

E-mail address:
sandra.anderson@sydney.edu.au

Exercise-Induced Bronchoconstriction
Celebrating 50 Years

Simon Godfrey, MD, PhD, FRCP, FRCPCH[a],*,
Kenneth D. Fitch, MD, MBBS, DSc (Hon), FACRM[b]

KEYWORDS

- Asthma • Exercise • Bronchoconstriction • Historical review • Airway drying
- Airway cooling • Refractory period • Athletes

The study of exercise-induced bronchospasm (EIB), alternatively called exercise-induced asthma (EIA), by many investigators over 50 years provides an outstanding example of how the techniques of classical physiology were applied in an attempt to determine the mechanisms underlying a troublesome clinical problem. Following the trail of this research in a more or less historical order enables the acknowledgment of the contributions of these investigators and follows the manner in which physiologic research was logically applied.

Perhaps the earliest description relating asthma to exercise was by Arataeus the Cappadocian around end of first century AD, as related by Brewis[1]:

If from running, gymnastic exercises, or any other work, the breathing become difficult, it is called Asthma ($\alpha\sigma\theta\mu\alpha$)

The initial classical description of EIB was published in 1717 in a book by Sir John Floyer,[2] himself an asthmatic, who wrote:

All violent exercise makes the asthmatic to breathe short—and if the exercise be continued it occasions a fit.

IS EIB A PROBLEM THAT NEEDS ATTENTION?

The practical implications of EIB were that 50 to 60 years ago, many asthmatics avoided exercise either from past personal experience of EIB or because parents restricted their children's involvement in sports and exercise. Such avoidance of

Funding Sources: Nil.
Conflicts of Interest: Nil.
[a] Hadassah Hebrew University, Jerusalem, Israel 91120; [b] School of Sports Science, Exercise and Health (M408), University of Western Australia, Crawley, Western Australia 6009, Australia
* Corresponding author. 156 Yehuda Street, Modiin 71724, Israel.
E-mail address: sgodfrey@netvision.net.il

physical activity was unfortunate because the lower a person's aerobic fitness, the higher the percentage of their maximum oxygen consumption ($Vo_{2\ max}$) that Is required to perform an exercise task.[3] Because the onset and severity of EIB is related to exercise intensity,[4] improved aerobic fitness allows asthmatics to undertake the same exercise at a lower percentage of their $Vo_{2\ max}$ and thus reduce the resultant EIB.[5] Conversely, in the very unfit, EIB is likely to appear even at low levels of exercise. However, although unaware of these principles of exercise physiology, there was a minority who had an alternative view that somehow exercise would benefit asthmatics and demonstrated this admirably. Theodore Roosevelt, who was President of the United States from 1901 to 1908, was a sickly child because of severe asthma. During adolescence, on advice from his physician, he undertook a program of vigorous exercise to grow into a fine athlete when he entered Harvard, only mildly inconvenienced by asthma.[6] Others would emulate Roosevelt and achieve great sporting success. One notable person was Dawn Fraser, from Australia, who commenced swimming "to lick asthma" and won the 100-m freestyle at 3 consecutive Olympic Games in 1956, 1960, and 1964, despite being troubled with asthma before her 1964 race.[7] Subsequently, the better understanding of the physiology of EIB and the benefit of a range of effective preventer medications has allowed those prone to EIB to achieve a level of fitness and enjoy a physical lifestyle comparable to their counterparts without EIB.[8]

1946–1970: EARLY MODERN ERA—ESTABLISHING BASIC FEATURES OF EIB

In 1946 Herxheimer[9] described 6 asthmatics with hyperventilation asthma, but in fact he meant hyperventilation induced by exercise. He made a most important observation, namely that the asthma (EIB) usually occurred after stopping exercise and not during the exercise.

A series of definitive studies of EIB were undertaken by a Liverpool, UK pediatrician, R.S. Jones,[10,11] and his colleagues from 1962 onwards,[12] which outlined almost all the important physiologic features. Brief exercise (running) of 1 to 2 minutes produced a rise in forced expiratory volume in 1 second (FEV_1) within 1 minute after stopping exercise, whereas prolonged exercise of 8 to 12 minutes produced a decrease in FEV_1, reaching its lowest level 1 to 5 minutes after exercise, which then rapidly returned to the resting level. **Fig. 1** shows an exercise challenge in a child with marked EIB in which there was a decrease of 55% in FEV_1 after exercise. They noted that the

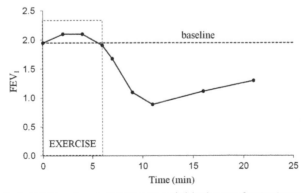

Fig. 1. Exercise-induced bronchoconstriction in a child who ran for 6 minutes on a treadmill. During the exercise there was a small rise in FEV_1. After stopping exercise, FEV_1 decreased to its lowest level 12 minutes after the end of exercise and then began to return to baseline.

intensity of exercise determined the severity of the response and that the EIB was minimized or abolished by the inhalation of a β-agonist, isoprenaline (isoproterenol). Subsequently Jones and colleagues[13] reported that the level of exercise had to be sufficient to produce moderate breathlessness. Even more importantly, they noted that in some subjects with a greater tendency to bronchoconstriction, the FEV_1 could decrease below the resting level even during the exercise. Thus EIB could occur during exercise—something that is discussed again later in this article. They also made an attempt to relate the exercise-induced changes in lung function and the clinical severity of asthma[14] and noted exercise performance could be limited because of bronchoconstriction during exercise.

About this time, McNeill and colleagues[15] showed that adults also developed EIB and found that with repeated exercise challenges on 6 occasions within 5 hours, the decrease in FEV_1 after exercise was less—the first recorded example of the development of refractoriness. Later, colleagues in North America also became interested in the diagnosis and treatment of EIB.[16,17]

1971–1976: STUDIES TO BETTER DEFINE THE STIMULUS OF EIB

Jones and colleagues[13] reported that they used free-range running as their stimulus for EIB because cycling was less effective, and a formal controlled study was undertaken by Anderson and colleagues[18] to compare treadmill running, free-range running, and cycling. They also found free-range running caused the most EIB but could not explain why this occurred. At the same time, Fitch and Morton[19] compared running, cycling, and swimming and found less EIA with swimming than running or cycling, whereas again running caused most EIB. The confusing situation in which exercise of different types but similar intensity caused different amounts of EIB resulted in Anderson and colleagues[20] writing a letter to the editor of the *British Medical Journal* stating, "Finally, we would like to repeat our earlier suggestion that the mechanism of exercise-induced asthma and the difference between the severe constriction due to running compared with the virtual absence during swimming may reflect neuromuscular differences in the types of exercise." How wrong we were! Various possibilities were considered related to hyperventilation versus exercise and changes in blood gases, which led to a vigorous exchange of letters in the *Lancet* by the major pioneers Herxheimer, Jones, and Anderson[9,21–27] but there was no convincing evidence to account for triggering EIB.

Although it had already been established that β-agonists could prevent EIB, presumably by a direct effect on bronchial smooth muscle, a new drug, sodium cromoglycate (cromolyn sodium), thought to block the release of mediators from mast cells, was shown by Davies[28] and Poppius and colleagues[29] to be effective in reducing the severity of EIB if inhaled before exercise but not if given once the attack had begun.[30] Oral glucorticosteroids, which by then were known to be highly effective in treating troublesome asthma, and the newly developed beclomethasone dipropionate taken by inhalation, were demonstrated to have little or no effect in preventing EIB in most asthmatics.[31] This latter outcome was so disappointing that it was more than a decade before a study of a newer inhaled corticosteroid, budesonide, was shown to be moderately effective in inhibiting EIB in children.[32] In more recent times the efficacy of regular use of inhaled corticosteroids in preventing EIB in both children and adults became well established.[33–35]

Silverman and Anderson[36] reported the results of carefully controlled studies to define the stimulus needed to obtain the maximal EIB response in children who ran or walked on a treadmill. EIB reached a maximum when the duration of exercise was 6 to 8 minutes and when the gradient of the treadmill was 10% to 15%, representing exercise at about 70% of maximum exercise performance. Exercise for longer periods or at steeper gradients produced no significant increase in bronchoconstriction. When tests were repeated at 2-hour intervals throughout the day, no significant diminution in EIB was found so that there was no refractoriness if the interval between challenges was 2 hours. In 1975 Anderson and colleagues[37] summarized what was known about EIB up to that time but were forced to admit that the mechanisms involved in the production of EIB remained largely unknown. Even something as apparently obvious as the site of action of a β-agonist in preventing EIB received a jolt when Anderson and colleagues[38] found that while an oral β-agonist, terbutaline, and an inhaled β-agonist, fenoterol, were equally effective as bronchodilators before and during exercise, only the inhaled drug prevented a post-exercise fall in lung function. There was still a decrease after the oral drug, albeit from a higher pre-exercise FEV_1 level. They suggested that perhaps the inhaled β-agonists had a second site of action "in or on the surface of the bronchial mucosa (perhaps the mast cell)."

The problems facing asthmatic athletes were reviewed by Fitch and Godfrey[39] in relation to the 1976 Olympic Games. They noted the ability of asthmatics to succeed especially in swimming and the effectiveness of $β_2$-agonists and sodium cromoglycate in preventing EIB. Although asthmatics could clearly now take part in sports with appropriate management, Fitch and colleagues[40] also showed that swim training for 5 months in children could improve physical fitness but, unfortunately, did not affect severity of EIB in response to running.

EXERCISE BRONCHIAL CHALLENGE IN NONASTHMATICS

In a foretaste of what would become of significant clinical interest much later, Day and Mearns[41] studied the response to exercise in 52 children with cystic fibrosis and found that most had increased bronchial lability or airway hyperresponsiveness (AHR), which was often manifest as bronchodilation rather than bronchoconstriction. This showed that AHR was not limited to asthmatics, although the pattern of response was different in that the response in asthmatics was mainly the decrease in lung function after exercise.

1976–1980: CLUES ABOUT THE MECHANISMS INVOLVED IN EIB START TO APPEAR

In 1976 Weinstein and colleagues[42] presented a paper at a meeting of the American Academy of Allergy in which he reported that 14 asthmatics exercising on a treadmill developed a mean decrease of FEV_1 of 29.5% breathing normal room air but only 13.5% breathing ultrasonically nebulized normal saline. He commented, "These results are similar to the results of others comparing the degree of bronchoconstriction occurring during treadmill running versus swimming. Bronchial drying may be an important mechanism in the development of EIA." A year later Bar-Or and colleagues[43] studied asthmatic children who exercised in a climate chamber. There was no effect of climate on resting lung function but breathing warm humid air virtually prevented EIB. Chen and Horton[44] obtained an identical result with asthmatic adults and suggested, "The results indicate that the primary stimulus for exercise-induced asthma may be heat loss and/or water loss from the airways during exercise." Strauss and colleagues[45] reported that subfreezing cold air had a negligible effect on lung function in asthmatics at rest but substantially increased the amount of EIB.

In several studies Deal and colleagues[46–48] measured respiratory heat exchange using inspired gas of differing temperature and humidity and showed a correlation between severity of EIB and respiratory heat loss. The emphasis in this study was on thermal load rather than drying of the airways and they concluded, "that the magnitude of exercise-induced asthma is directly proportional to the thermal load placed on the airways and that this reaction is quantifiable in terms of respiratory heat exchange." Subsequently they demonstrated that breathing cold dry air actually lowered esophageal temperature during exercise. They also showed that asthmatics could get bronchoconstriction with isocapnic hyperventilation (hyperventilation induced bronchoconstriction, HIB) similar to that seen with exercise and that it responded similarly to ambient conditions and severity of hyperventilation.

At this time there began a long controversy as to the relative importance of cooling and drying of the airways in the triggering of EIB. That both the thermal effects on the vasculature and the osmotic effects on mediator release could occur separately or together to enhance one another was discussed in depth much later by Anderson and Daviskas.[49]

The next clue was the refractory period. Although a study in 1966 had noted reduced EIB with repeated exercise,[15] it was 12 years later that Edmonds and colleagues[50] undertook a formal study and showed that an episode of EIB was followed by a refractory period and that the response in the second of a pair of challenges decreased as the interval between them decreased. When exercise challenge tests at varying metabolic loads were followed after 30 minutes by tests at a constant load, the severity of EIB in the constant load challenge decreased in proportion to the load in the first challenge of each pair. They commented that, "These results were compatible with the suggestion that the development of EIB requires the release of a stored mediator or enzyme precursor." Another clue was provided by Schnall and Landau,[51] who showed that short warm-up sprints could prevent EIB in a subsequent 6-minute run. Not everyone agreed with this suggestion and Deal and colleagues[52] measured arterial histamine and neutrophil chemotactic activity during hyperventilation, which they considered was the same thing as exercise and found no changes in either activity. They concluded that mediators derived from mast cells were not involved in EIB. They chose to dismiss refractory period data because there could have been persistent sympatho-adrenal activity between closely spaced challenges. In other words, the secretion of adrenaline during the first exercise challenge could have persisted and reduced the response in the second. Even so, a lot of similarities were found between EIB and HIB, including refractoriness and cross-refractoriness between the 2 types of challenge,[53,54] making the sympatho-adrenal theory of refractoriness very unlikely. The similarities led investigators to develop a protocol for using voluntary hyperpnea with dry air containing 4.9% CO_2 as a surrogate for exercise to identify EIB in defense force recruits. This protocol is still widely used for identifying EIB in athletes.[55]

Both knowledge of the ameliorating effect of humidity and the development of refractoriness to repeated exercise were put into practice as nonpharmacologic methods of ameliorating EIB. Warm-up exercises, whether continuous or intermittent, were shown to result in modest reductions of EIB.[56,57] The use of face masks to humidify and heat the inspired air in an attempt to attenuate EIB was investigated in 1980 and did produce modest protection.[58,59]

1981–1985 AND THEN OSMOLARITY AS A STIMULUS FOR EIB AND SOME OTHER OBSERVATIONS

Exploring a different type of challenge, Schoeffel and colleagues[60] in Anderson's laboratory found that an attack of asthma could be provoked in asthmatics but not in normal subjects by having them breathe an ultrasonically nebulized aerosol, which was either hypertonic or hypotonic, but not by breathing an isotonic aerosol. Later when Anderson and colleagues[61] measured respiratory heat and water loss in young asthmatics exercising under various ambient conditions, they showed that EIB became worse as the water content of the inspired air was reduced, although some subjects experienced EIB, albeit to a lesser degree, when breathing warm humid air. The authors postulated that water loss from the airways during exercise may induce a change in osmolarity similar to that observed with the inhalation of hypertonic saline. Moreover, at the high levels of ventilation during exercise with "hot wet" air, there could be a net gain in water in the airways in some patients leading to a reduction in osmolarity of the respiratory tract fluid. Anderson and colleagues[61] postulated "A unifying hypothesis for the bronchoconstricting effect from water gain and water loss from the airways may be a change in the tonicity of the fluid lining the respiratory tract." This hypothesis emphasized for the first time, the very small volume of fluid in the generations of airways involved in conditioning the inspired air, and the capacity for the osmolarity of this small volume to change rapidly.[62]

In 1982 Bar-Yishay and colleagues[63] finally tackled the problem of swimming versus running as the challenge for EIB by having children run and swim while breathing either dry or humid air. Although the EIB was less under both conditions with swimming, nevertheless the children had substantial EIB swimming while breathing dry air and so the difference between running and swimming in earlier studies must have been climatic.

Despite an earlier study that failed to detect any mediator release during HIB,[52] neutrophil chemotactic factor (NCF) was shown by Lee and colleagues[64] to be released during exercise in asthmatics but not in normal subjects. The level peaked 10 minutes after exercise and returned to baseline by 1 hour and paralleled the decrease in lung function. Later they demonstrated that NCF was liberated in asthmatics breathing cold dry air but not warm humid air[65] and that NCF was also liberated in hyperventilation-induced asthma.[66] The present authors and many others were all very excited by these observations but, as it is now known, NCF is almost certainly interlukin-8 and not a mast cell–liberated mediator at all!

By placing a probe in a segment of the right lower lobe in normal subjects who hyperventilated, McFadden and colleagues[67] showed that the airways can get very cold when breathing cold air. In a further study in 1985[68] using multiple probes, they showed that the intrathoracic and intrapulmonary airways can undergo profound thermal changes that extend into the periphery of the lung.

1986–1990: A NEW HYPOTHESIS—REWARMING AND REACTIVE HYPEREMIA IS THE TRIGGER FOR EIB

In 1986 McFadden and colleagues[69] reported that the temperature of the air breathed on rewarming after the airways were cooled during exercise affected the severity of EIB such that the quicker the rewarming, the worse the EIB, which led them to postulate that perhaps the trigger for EIB was a type of reactive hyperemia of the airway vasculature. "This in turn could result in luminal narrowing from vascular engorgement and edema in the mucosa and submucosa."[69] By contrast, however, Hahn and colleagues[70] found that the airway response to exercise was not significantly different when inspired air temperature varied considerably provided the amount of water required to saturate the inspired air remained the same. They concluded that it was the osmotic and not the cooling effects induced by the vaporization of water that was the more important factor determining EIB. Moreover, Smith and colleagues[71] also undertook a rapid rewarming study and were unable to show any difference in the severity of EIB in relation to the rate of rewarming. Continuing the "battle" over the trigger for EIB, Gilbert and colleagues[72] presented calculations showing that the fluid loss from the airways in relation to the amount available during exercise would not be enough to cause a change in osmolarity. These conflicting hypotheses, drying-osmolarity versus cooling-hyperemia, were summarized in detail by Anderson in 1989[73] and Anderson and colleagues in 1992,[74] who presented strong arguments against the hyperemia hypothesis and in favor of the osmolar hypothesis. Suffice to say that it was and remains very difficult for the hyperemia hypothesis to explain the appearance of EIB in many subjects during exercise while the airways were still cold and when no rewarming had occurred, nor why the duration of exercise affects the severity of EIB. It also does not explain why severe EIB can occur when hot dry air is inspired during exercise and the airways do not cool abnormally.[75]

ANOTHER POSSIBLE PATHWAY TO EXPLAIN REFRACTORINESS

Although the release of a chemical mediator in response to a trigger was attractive to many as the intermediary pathway to explain why EIB exhibits refractoriness, there were several problematic observations. Some years ago Ben Dov and colleagues[76] were surprised to find refractoriness to EIB in subjects exercising and breathing cold, dry air following a previous exercise challenge breathing warm, humid air, which itself did not provoke EIB. In fact, such an observation can be deduced from an earlier study by Henriksen and colleagues[77] and was repeated in 1990 with exactly the same results by Wilson and colleagues.[78] Interestingly NCF did not show any reduction in release by exercise when the subject was refractory[79] but it is now known that it is not a mediator. A totally new light on the refractoriness issue was shed by O'Byrne and colleagues[80] in 1986 and later by others who showed that the prostaglandin inhibitor, indomethacin, could prevent the appearance of refractoriness to EIB and osmotically induced bronchospasm but not to HIB,[81,82] which suggests that refractoriness, at least to exercise and hyposmolar challenges, is due to the release of an inhibitory prostaglandin, the effect of which persists for 30 to 60 minutes or so after the initial challenge and whose release does not require that the initial challenge causes actual bronchoconstriction. However, not everyone agreed with the observation of refractoriness after a challenge that did not provoke asthma. Studies by Hahn and colleagues[83] using exercise and by Bar-Yishay and colleagues[53] using hyperventilation failed to demonstrate refractoriness after such challenges. The 3 major mediators considered important in EIB were histamine, prostaglandins, and leukotrienes. Histamine and prostaglandins were implicated in EIB, however, by the finding that alone or in combination an antihistamine terfenadine and a prostaglandin synthetase inhibitor, flurbiprofen, gave significant protection from EIB.[84] One of the first studies to investigate concentrations of all 3 mediators used 5 minutes of dry air hyperpnea at 22°C as the stimulus and measured changes in bronchoalveolar lavage fluid. They showed significant increases in levels of leukotriene B4 and SRS-A (a mixture of other leukotrienes).[85] As with the earlier studies, some, but not all, subjects had increases in prostaglandin D2 and histamine levels. It is still a mystery as to what causes refractoriness to EIB and a challenge for a new generation of investigators.

1991–1995: EXERCISE CHALLENGE HAS A DIFFERENTIAL DIAGNOSTIC ROLE

In 1991 Godfrey and colleagues[86] began to explore the use of bronchial challenges as an aid in the differential diagnosis of pediatric lung diseases. Bronchial provocation challenges with exercise and methacholine were performed on the same day or within a short interval in 52 children with asthma, 22 with other types of chronic lung disease (including cystic fibrosis), and 19 control subjects with no evidence of chronic lung disease. In the methacholine challenges 94% of patients with asthma and 82% of patients with chronic lung disease responded abnormally. However, in the exercise challenges 79% of asthmatic patients but none of those with chronic lung disease responded abnormally. Thus the response to the 2 types of challenge was able to distinguish asthma from other types of chronic lung disease in children. The same investigators[87] compared the responses of asthmatic children, children with chronic obstructive pulmonary disease (COPD), and normal controls, to challenges by exercise, by the inhalation of methacholine (thought to act directly on bronchial smooth muscle), and by the inhalation of adenosine 5′-monophosphate (AMP), thought to act indirectly by liberating mediators. They found the direct challenge by methacholine distinguished both asthma and pediatric COPD from controls with a sensitivity of 82% to 92%, but did not distinguish between asthma and pediatric COPD. In contrast, both exercise and AMP distinguished asthma from controls with a sensitivity and specificity of 84% to 98% but they also distinguished asthma from pediatric COPD with a sensitivity and specificity of 85% to 90%. The similarity of the exercise and AMP results also suggested that exercise acted through a mediator-related intermediary pathway like that activated by AMP.

AN UPDATED REVIEW OF EIB

In 1993 Godfrey and Bar-Yishay[88] updated the review of EIB published in 1975.[37] They concluded that after 18 years of exciting research their original conclusion still stood with the addition of one word—complete. "There is as yet no complete explanation for the mechanism of exercise-induced asthma, but it is a tool of potentially great value for research into the physiology and treatment of clinical asthma."

A possible further piece of the jigsaw puzzle came to light when Manning and colleagues[89] undertook crossover challenges with exercise and the leukotriene D$_4$ (LTD4) with and without flurbiprofen (a prostaglandin synthetase inhibitor). They found refractoriness occurred with all types of paired challenges and was reduced by flurbiprofen in all cases. They proposed that EIB was partly due to release of LTD4 and this in turn released an inhibitory prostaglandin. Subsequently, Reiss and colleagues[90] showed that montelukast, a potent cysteinyl leukotriene receptor antagonist, attenuated EIB, providing further evidence of the role of leukotrienes in the pathogenesis of EIB.

1999: WHEN IS EIB REALLY ABNORMAL EIB?

Throughout most of the time that EIB has been studied, different investigators have chosen different criteria to define a decrease in lung function, which was considered a positive asthmatic response. In almost all cases there was no serious attempt to use statistical techniques to define the cutoff between a normal and an asthmatic response. The same applied to bronchial challenges by other means, such as an inhalation challenge by methacholine. In 1999 Godfrey and colleagues[91] addressed this problem by extracting much data from published reports of the response of young normal subjects and asthmatics to challenges with exercise or methacholine. Using receiver operating characteristic curves, they found that the optimal cutoff point to distinguish asthmatics from normal subjects was a decrease in FEV$_1$ after exercise of 13%, with a sensitivity of 63% and a specificity of 94%. For inhalation challenges, the optimal cutoff point for the dose of methacholine (or histamine) causing a 20% decrease in FEV$_1$ was 6.6 μm, with a sensitivity of 92% and a specificity of 89%. Unfortunately, despite the availability of this evidence, many studies continue to be reported using arbitrary criteria to define a positive response and even the Guidelines for Methacholine and Exercise Challenges published by the American Thoracic Society[92] state that "A decrease below 90% of the baseline FEV_1 (ie, a 10% decrease) is a generally accepted abnormal response. Some authors suggest a value of 15% is more diagnostic of EIB, particularly if exercise has been performed in the field."

SO WHAT MORE HAS BEEN LEARNED ABOUT EIB SINCE THEN, IN THE PAST FEW YEARS?

To be honest, despite the impressive amount of information accumulated by many talented investigators, there still remains much for future generations to sort out.

- Although there is a general consensus that both drying and cooling are involved in the triggering of EIB, how this occurs is still uncertain and other articles in this series discuss this important issue.
- It is still not known for sure whether mediators are liberated by the trigger and, if so, what mediators are involved.
- It is still not known for sure what makes an asthmatic refractory to EIB shortly after a previous attack.

Work on these and other aspects of EIB has continued and an interesting new aspect of the subject has opened up with competitive athletes giving us much more to think about.

1993–2012: WINTER AND SUMMER ATHLETES AND ASTHMA/AHR

The finding of a high prevalence of bronchial hyperresponsiveness in athletes was reported in 1986 and many studies followed. Weiler and colleagues[93] documented a positive response to methacholine challenge in 76 of 151 young adult footballers, although only 12% admitted to a history of asthma. In 1993 Larsson and colleagues[94] noted a high prevalence of asthma in cross-country skiers and undertook methacholine challenges in 42 skiers and 29 controls. No less that 33 skiers had either asthma symptoms or AHR compared with just one in the control group, raising the question of the relationship between exercise and asthma, although inspiring cold air was considered to be a major factor. However, a later study by Helenius and colleagues[95] identified a higher prevalence of physician-diagnosed asthma in elite long-distance Finnish runners compared with their counterparts who participated in speed and power events. This discrepancy seemed to incriminate years of endurance exercise training as a factor, actually provoking AHR and thus being prone to EIB. In time, this would be considered to be due to an inability to condition large volumes of inspired air during years of endurance training causing airway injury.[96] A high prevalence of EIB was found by Mannix and colleagues[97] among competitive ice skaters. Other indoor athletes, such as ice hockey players, were also reported to be at risk and initially considered to be at risk because of the lower air temperatures in ice rinks,[98] but later inhaling particulate matter from diesel-powered ice resurfacers was found as the incriminating factor.[99]

When the International Olympic Committee demanded in 2001 that athletes who wished to use an inhaled β-2 agonist (IBA) at the Olympic Games must confirm asthma/AHR by either a positive bronchodilator or a positive bronchial provocation test,[100] this resulted in the accumulation of considerable data over the next 5 Olympic Games.[101,102] Not only did it confirm that athletes engaging in endurance training had a higher prevalence of asthma/AHR and were approved to use IBA but also that many did not have any history of childhood asthma with their onset of asthma/AHR being after the age of 16 years. One additional and perhaps surprising finding was that athletes who had been approved to use IBA at Olympic Games actually outperformed their rivals. The reason was unclear because IBAs do not enhance performance. It is postulated that these athletes train harder and longer and thus became superior athletes, but in doing so, sustain more airway injury because they are unable to condition the increased volumes of inspired air. However, what occurs to the airways of these endurance trained athletes when they cease training? There is some anecdotal evidence that they may lose their AHR and proneness to EIB and this has been reported to occur in Finnish swimmers 5 years into their retirement[103]; however, more research is necessary to confirm this outcome.

In 2010 Sue-Chu and colleagues[104] studied bronchial responsiveness in 58 elite cross-country skiers to several challenges including eucapnic hyperventilation, exercise, methacholine, AMP, and mannitol. They found that although 25 (43%) skiers had hyperresponsiveness, in the large majority the hyperresponsiveness was to methacholine, which according to the work discussed earlier is relatively nonspecific.[87] Only 5 and 3 subjects, respectively, were hyperresponsive to AMP and mannitol, which are much more specific for asthma. Even more surprising, methacholine hyperresponsiveness was more prevalent in subjects without asthmalike symptoms. They concluded that the low prevalence of hyperresponsiveness to indirect stimuli (exercise, hyperventilation, AMP, and mannitol) may suggest differences in the pathogenesis of methacholine hyperresponsiveness between elite skiers and nonathletes. In a review of asthma and airway hyperresponsiveness in Olympic athletes, Fitch suggested that the increased incidence of abnormal responses was likely to have been a consequence of their training.[105] Some might suggest that the symptoms in most athletes are due to a type of airway trauma and not to genetically based atopic allergic asthma, which is the common pattern seen in children and young adults.

SUMMARY

Therefore, for over 50 years, from the first modern studies in 1946, a large number of investigators have gradually pieced together most, but not all, of the pathophysiologic pathways involved in EIB. The story of EIB surely provides a case for the need to understand and apply classical physiology in this era of molecular genetics. As a consequence of this research, the burden of EIB has largely been removed from asthmatics of all ages, who can now lead much more normal lives.

REFERENCES

1. Brewis RA. Classic papers in asthma. London: Science Press Limited; 1990.
2. Floyer SJ. A treatise of the asthma. London: R. Wilkin & W. Innis; 1698.
3. Astrand PO, Rodahl K. Textbook of work physiology. New York: McGraw Hill; 1970.
4. Carlsson E, Engh G, Mork M. Exercise-induced bronchoconstriction depends on exercise load. Respir Med 2000;94:750–5.
5. Henriksen JM, Nielsen TT. Effect of physical training on exercise-induced bronchoconstriction. Acta Paediatr Scand 1983;72:31–6.
6. Szanton VL. Theodore Roosevelt, the asthmatic. Ann Allergy 1969;27:485–9.
7. Frazer D. Gold medal girl. Melbourne (Australia): Landsdowne; 1965.
8. Fitch KD. Pharmacotherapy for exercise-induced asthma: allowing normal levels of activity and sport. Expert Rev Clin Pharmacol 2010;3:139–52.
9. Herxheimer H. Hyperventilation asthma. Lancet 1946;1:83–7.
10. Jones RS, Buston MH, Wharton MJ. The effect of exercise on ventilatory function in the child with asthma. Br J Dis Chest 1962;56:78–86.

11. Jones RH, Jones RS. Ventilatory capacity in young adults with a history of asthma in childhood. Br Med J 1966;2:976–8.
12. Blackhall M. Ventilatory function in subjects with childhood asthma who have become symptom free. Arch Dis Child 1970;45:363–6.
13. Jones RS, Wharton MJ, Buston MH. The place of physical exercise and bronchodilator drugs in the assessment of the asthmatic child. Arch Dis Child 1963;38:539–45.
14. Jones RS. Assessment of respiratory function in the asthmatic child. Br Med J 1966;2:972–5.
15. McNeill RS, Nairn JR, Millar JS, et al. Exercise induced asthma. Q J Med 1966; 35:55–67.
16. Sly RM, Heimlich EM, Busser RJ, et al. Exercise induced bronchospasm: effect of adrenergic or cholinergic blockade. J Allergy 1967;40:93–9.
17. Pierson WE, Bierman CW, Stamm SJ. Cycloergometer induced bronchospasm. J Allergy 1969;43:136–44.
18. Anderson SD, Connolly NM, Godfrey S. Comparison of bronchoconstriction induced by cycling and running. Thorax 1971;26:396–401.
19. Fitch KD, Morton AR. Specificity of exercise-induced asthma. Br Med J 1971;4: 577–81.
20. Anderson SD, Silverman M, Tai E, et al. Specificity of exercise in exercise-induced asthma. Br Med J 1971;4:814–5.
21. Herxheimer H. Exercise asthma. Lancet 1972;1:436–7.
22. Beaudry PH, Wise MB, Seely JE. Respiratory gas exchange at rest and during exercise in normal and asthmatic children. Am Rev Respir Dis 1967;95: 248–54.
23. Seaton A, Davies G, Gaziano D, et al. Exercise induced asthma. Br Med J 1969; 3:556–8.
24. Katz RM, Whipp BJ, Heimlich EM, et al. Exercise induced bronchospasm, ventilation and blood gases in asthmatic children. J Allergy 1971;47:148–58.
25. Anderson SD, Silverman M, Walker SR. Metabolic and ventilatory changes in asthmatic patients during and after exercise. Thorax 1972;27:718–25.
26. Jones RS, Godfrey S, Silverman M, et al. Exercise asthma. Lancet 1972;1:533.
27. Silverman M, Anderson SD, Walker SR. Metabolic changes preceding exercise-induced bronchoconstriction. Br Med J 1972;1:207–9.
28. Davies SE. The effect of disodium cromoglycate on exercise-induced asthma. Br Med J 1968;3:593–4.
29. Poppius H, Muittari A, Kreus KE, et al. Exercise induced asthma and disodium cromoglycate. Br Med J 1970;4:337–9.
30. Silverman M, Andrea T. Time course of effect of disodium cromoglycate on exercise-induced asthma. Arch Dis Child 1972;47:419–22.
31. Konig P, Jaffe P, Godfrey S. Effect of corticosteroids on exercise-induced asthma. J Allergy Clin Immunol 1974;54:14–9.
32. Henriksen JM, Dahl R. Effects of inhaled budesonide alone and in combination with low dose terbutaline in children with exercise-induced asthma. Am Rev Respir Dis 1983;128:993–7.
33. Hofstra WB, Sterk PJ, Neijens HJ, et al. Prolonged recovery from exercise-induced asthma with increasing age in childhood. Pediatr Pulmonol 1995;20: 177–83.
34. Jonasson G, Carlsen KH, Hultquist C. Low-dose budesonide improves exercise-induced bronchospasm in schoolchildren. Pediatr Allergy Immunol 2000;11: 120–5.

35. Subbarao P, Duong M, Adelroth E, et al. Effect of ciclesonide dose and duration of therapy on exercise-induced bronchoconstriction in patients with asthma. J Allergy Clin Immunol 2006;117:1008–13.
36. Silverman M, Anderson SD. Standardization of exercise tests in asthmatic children. Arch Dis Child 1972;47:882–9.
37. Anderson SD, Silverman M, Konig P, et al. Exercise-induced asthma. Br J Dis Chest 1975;69:1–39.
38. Anderson SD, Rozea PJ, Dolton R, et al. Inhaled and oral bronchodilator therapy in exercise induced asthma. Aust N Z J Med 1975;5:544–50.
39. Fitch KD, Godfrey S. Asthma and athletic performance. JAMA 1976;236:152–7.
40. Fitch KD, Morton AR, Blanksby BA. Effects of swimming training on children with asthma. Arch Dis Child 1976;51:190–4.
41. Day G, Mearns MB. Bronchial lability in cystic fibrosis. Arch Dis Child 1973;48: 355–9.
42. Weinstein RE, Anderson JA, Kvale P, et al. Effects of humidification on exercise-induced asthma (EIA). J Allergy Clin Immunol 1976;57:250–1.
43. Bar-Or O, Neuman I, Dotan R. Effects of dry and humid climates on exercise-induced asthma in children and adolescents. J Allergy Clin Immunol 1977;60: 163–8.
44. Chen WY, Horton DJ. Heat and water loss from the airways and exercise-induced asthma. Respiration 1977;34:305–13.
45. Strauss RH, McFadden ER, Ingram RH, et al. Enhancement of exercise-induced asthma by cold air. N Engl J Med 1977;297:743–7.
46. Deal EC, McFadden ER, Ingram RH, et al. Role of respiratory heat exchange in production of exercise-induced asthma. J Appl Physiol 1979;46:467–75.
47. Deal EC, McFadden ER, Ingram RH, et al. Esophageal temperature during exercise in asthmatic and non-asthmatic subjects. J Appl Physiol 1979;46: 484–90.
48. Deal EC, McFadden ER, Ingram RH, et al. Hyperpnea and heat flux: initial reaction sequence in exercise-induced asthma. J Appl Physiol 1979;46:476–83.
49. Anderson SD, Daviskas E. The mechanism of exercise-induced asthma is.... J Allergy Clin Immunol 2000;106:453–9.
50. Edmunds AT, Tooley M, Godfrey S. The refractory period after exercise-induced asthma: its duration and relation to the severity of exercise. Am Rev Respir Dis 1978;117:247–54.
51. Schnall RP, Landau LI. The protective effects of short sprints in exercise induced asthma. Thorax 1980;35:828–32.
52. Deal EC, Wasserman SI, Soter NA, et al. Evaluation of role played by mediators of immediate hypersensitivity in exercise-induced asthma. J Clin Invest 1980;65: 659–65.
53. Bar-Yishay E, Ben Dov I, Godfrey S. Refractory period after hyperventilation-induced asthma. Am Rev Respir Dis 1983;127:572–4.
54. Ben Dov I, Gur I, Bar-Yishay E, et al. Refractory period following induced asthma: contributions of exercise and isocapnic hyperventilation. Thorax 1983; 38:849–53.
55. Phillips YY, Jaeger JJ, Laube BL, et al. Eucapnic voluntary hyperventilation of compressed gas mixture. A simple system for bronchial challenge by respiratory heat loss. Am Rev Respir Dis 1985;131:31–5.
56. Reiff DB, Choudry NB, Pride NB, et al. The effect of prolonged submaximal warm-up exercise on exercise-induced asthma. Am Rev Respir Dis 1989;139: 479–84.

57. McKenzie DC, McLuckie SL, Stirling DR. The protective effects of continuous and interval exercise in athletes with exercise-induced asthma. Med Sci Sports Exerc 1994;26:951–6.
58. Brenner AM, Weiser PC, Krogh LA, et al. Effectiveness of a portable face mask in attenuating exercise-induced asthma. JAMA 1980;244:2196–8.
59. Schachter EN, Lee M, Gerhard H, et al. A non-pharmacologic approach to the treatment of exercise-induced bronchospasm. Yale J Biol Med 1980;53:485–96.
60. Schoeffel RE, Anderson SD, Altounyan RE. Bronchial hyperreactivity in response to inhalation of ultrasonically nebulised solutions of distilled water and saline. Br Med J 1981;282:1285–7.
61. Anderson SD, Schoeffel RE, Follet R, et al. Sensitivity to heat and water loss at rest and during exercise in asthmatic patients. Eur J Respir Dis 1982;63: 459–571.
62. Anderson SD. Is there a unifying hypothesis for exercise-induced asthma. J Allergy Clin Immunol 1984;73:660–5.
63. Bar-Yishay E, Gur I, Inbar O, et al. Differences between swimming and running as stimuli for exercise- induced asthma. Eur J Appl Physiol 1982;48:387–97.
64. Lee TH, Nagy L, Nakagura T, et al. Identification and partial characterization of an exercise-induced neutrophil chemotatic factor in bronchial asthma. J Clin Invest 1982;69:889–99.
65. Lee TH, Assoufi BK, Kay AB. The link between exercise, respiratory heat exchange, and the mast cell in bronchial asthma. Lancet 1983;1:520–2.
66. Nagakura T, Lee TH, Assoufi BK, et al. Neutrophil chemotactic factor in exercise- and hyperventilation-induced asthma. Am Rev Respir Dis 1983;126:294–6.
67. McFadden ER, Denison DM, Waller JF, et al. Direct recordings of the temperatures in the tracheobronchial tree in normal man. J Clin Invest 1982;69:700–5.
68. McFadden ER, Pichurko BM, Bowman HF, et al. Thermal mapping of the airways in humans. J Appl Physiol 1985;58:564–70.
69. McFadden ER, Lenner KA, Strohl KP. Postexertional airway rewarming and thermally induced asthma. New insights into pathophysiology and possible pathogenesis. J Clin Invest 1986;78:18–25.
70. Hahn A, Anderson SD, Morton AR, et al. A reinterpretation of the effect of temperature and water content of the inspired air in exercise-induced asthma. Am Rev Respir Dis 1984;130:575–9.
71. Smith CM, Anderson SD, Walsh S, et al. An investigation of the effects of heat and water exchange in the recovery period after exercise in children with asthma. Am Rev Respir Dis 1989;140:598–605.
72. Gilbert IA, Fouke JM, McFadden ER. Heat and water flux in the intrathoracic airways and exercise-induced asthma. J Appl Physiol 1987;63:1681–91.
73. Anderson SD, Daviskas E, Smith CM. Exercise-induced asthma: a difference in opinion regarding the stimulus. Allergy Proc 1989;10:215–26.
74. Anderson SD, Daviskas E. The airway microvasculature and exercise induced asthma. Thorax 1992;47:748–52.
75. Anderson SD, Schoeffel RE, Black JL, et al. Airway cooling as the stimulus to exercise-induced asthma - a re-evaluation. Eur J Respir Dis 1985;67:20–30.
76. Ben Dov I, Bar-Yishay E, Godfrey S. Refractory period after exercise-induced asthma unexplained by respiratory heat loss. Am Rev Respir Dis 1982;125: 530–4.
77. Henriksen JM, Dahl R, Lundquist GR. Influence of relative humidity and repeated exercise on exercise-induced bronchoconstriction. Allergy 1981;36: 463–70.

78. Wilson BA, Bar-Or O, Seed LG. Effects of humid air breathing during arm or treadmill exercise on exercise-induced bronchoconstriction and refractoriness. Am Rev Respir Dis 1990;142:349–52.
79. Belcher NG, Murdoch RD, Dalton N, et al. A comparison of mediator and catecholamine release between exercise- and hypertonic saline-induced asthma. Am Rev Respir Dis 1988;137:1026–32.
80. O'Byrne PM, Jones GM. The effect of indomethecin on exercise-induced bronchoconstriction and refractoriness after exercise. Am Rev Respir Dis 1986;134:69–72.
81. Margolskee DJ, Bigby BG, Boushey HA. Indomethecin blocks airway tolerance to repetitive exercise but not to eucapnic hyperpnea in asthmatic subjects. Am Rev Respir Dis 1988;137:842–6.
82. Mattoli S, Foresi A, Corbo GM, et al. The effect of indomethacin on the refractory period occurring after the inhalation of ultrasonically nebulised distilled water. J Allergy Clin Immunol 1987;79:678–83.
83. Hahn AG, Nogrady SG, Burton GR, et al. Absence of refractoriness in asthmatic subjects after exercise with warm, humid inspirate. Thorax 1985;40:418–21.
84. Finnerty JP, Holgate ST. Evidence for the roles of histamine and prostaglandins as mediators in exercise-induced asthma: the inhibitory effect of terfenadine and flurbiprofen alone and in combination. Eur Respir J 1990;3:540–7.
85. Pliss LB, Ingenito EP, Ingram RH Jr, et al. Assessment of bronchoalveolar cell and mediator response to isocapnic hyperpnea in asthma. Am J Respir Crit Care Med 1990;142:73–8.
86. Godfrey S, Springer C, Noviski N, et al. Exercise but not methacholine differentiates asthma from chronic lung disease in children. Thorax 1991;46:488–92.
87. Avital A, Springer C, Bar-Yishay E, et al. Adenosine, methacholine, and exercise challenges in children with asthma or paediatric chronic obstructive pulmonary disease. Thorax 1995;50:511–6.
88. Godfrey S, Bar-Yishay E. Exercised-induced asthma revisited. Respir Med 1993;87:331–44.
89. Manning PJ, Watson RM, O'Byrne PM. Exercise-induced refractoriness in asthmatic subjects involves leukotriene and prostaglandin interdependent mechanisms. Am Rev Respir Dis 1993;148:950–4.
90. Reiss TF, Hill JB, Harman E, et al. Increased urinary excretion of LTE4 after exercise and attenuation of exercise-induced bronchospasm by montelukast, a cysteinyl leukotriene receptor antagonist. Thorax 1997;52:1030–5.
91. Godfrey S, Springer C, Bar-Yishay E, et al. Cut-off points defining normal and asthmatic bronchial reactivity to exercise and inhalation challenges in children and young adults. Eur Respir J 1999;14:659–68.
92. Crapo RO, Casaburi R, Coates AL, et al. Guidelines for methacholine and exercise challenge testing-1999. Am J Respir Crit Care Med 2000;161:309–29.
93. Weiler JM, Metzger WJ, Donnelly AL, et al. Prevalence of bronchial hyperresponsiveness in highly trained athletes. Chest 1986;90:23–8.
94. Larsson K, Ohlson P, Larsson L, et al. High prevalence of asthma in cross country skiers. Br Med J 1993;307:1326–9.
95. Helenius IJ, Tikkanen HO, Haahtela T. Association between type of training and risk of asthma in elite athletes. Thorax 1997;52:157–60.
96. Anderson SD, Kippelen P. Airway injury as a mechanism for exercise-induced bronchoconstriction in elite athletes. J Allergy Clin Immunol 2008;122:225–35.
97. Mannix ET, Farber MO, Palange P, et al. Exercise-induced asthma in figure skaters. Chest 1996;109:312–5.

98. Leuppi JD, Kuhn M, Comminot C, et al. High prevalence of bronchial hyperresponsiveness and asthma in ice hockey players. Eur Respir J 1998;12:13–6.
99. Rundell KW. Pulmonary function decay in women ice hockey players: is there a relationship to ice rink air quality? Inhal Toxicol 2004;16:117–23.
100. Anderson SD, Fitch K, Perry CP, et al. Responses to bronchial challenge submitted for approval to use inhaled beta2-agonists before an event at the 2002 Winter Olympics. J Allergy Clin Immunol 2003;111:45–50.
101. Anderson SD, Sue-Chu M, Perry CP, et al. Bronchial challenges in athletes applying to inhale a beta2-agonist at the 2004 Summer Olympics. J Allergy Clin Immunol 2006;117:767–73.
102. Fitch KD, Sue-Chu M, Anderson SD, et al. Asthma and the elite athlete: summary of the International Olympic Committee's consensus conference, Lausanne, Switzerland, January 22-24, 2008. J Allergy Clin Immunol 2008;122: 254–60, 260.e1–7.
103. Helenius I, Rytila P, Sarna S, et al. Effect of continuing or finishing high-level sports on airway inflammation, bronchial hyperresponsiveness, and asthma: a 5-year prospective follow-up study of 42 highly trained swimmers. J Allergy Clin Immunol 2002;109:962–8.
104. Sue-Chu M, Brannan JD, Anderson SD, et al. Airway hyperresponsiveness to methacholine, adenosine 5-monophosphate, mannitol, eucapnic voluntary hyperpnoea and field exercise challenge in elite cross-country skiers. Br J Sports Med 2010;44:827–32.
105. Fitch KD. An overview of asthma and airway hyper-responsiveness in Olympic athletes. Br J Sports Med 2012;46:413–6.

Pathogenesis of Exercise-Induced Bronchoconstriction

Pascale Kippelen, PhD[a],*, Sandra D. Anderson, PhD, DSc, MD(Hon)[b]

KEYWORDS

- Hyperpnoea • Osmotic stress • Thermal stress • Epithelial injury
- Airway inflammation

KEY POINTS

- The increased ventilatory demand associated with exercise is a major determinant in exercise-induced bronchoconstriction (EIB).
- In susceptible individuals, the drying and cooling of the intrathoracic airways secondary to increased ventilatory flow trigger a cascade of events that ultimately leads to airway narrowing.
- This cascade of events may include epithelial injury, inflammatory mediator release, vasculature hyperemia, and/or sensory nerve activation.
- A dysfunctional airway epithelium, either inherited or acquired, is thought central in the long-term development or progression of EIB.
- Environmental factors interacting with genetic predispositions modulate the airway response to exercise and contribute to the complex nature and pathogenesis of EIB.

INTRODUCTION

Exercise-induced bronchoconstriction (EIB) is defined as a transient airway narrowing that occurs shortly after strenuous exercise. EIB is highly prevalent in individuals with clinical asthma but can also occur in otherwise healthy individuals. Because exercise is unavoidable at times, and sudden bronchoconstriction triggered by exercise can be fatal,[1] understanding the mechanisms for EIB is a prerequisite for developing effective strategies for its prevention and treatment.

While exercise is recognized as a potent trigger for bronchoconstriction, it is not the exercise per se that is directly responsible for the airway narrowing, but rather the hyperpnoea associated with it. When people exercise, the ventilatory demand

Funding Sources: None.
Conflict of Interest: None.
[a] Centre for Sports Medicine & Human Performance, Brunel University, Uxbridge, Middlesex UB8 3PH, UK; [b] Department of Respiratory and Sleep Medicine, Royal Prince Alfred Hospital, Camperdown, New South Wales 2050, Australia
* Corresponding author.
E-mail address: pascale.kippelen@brunel.ac.uk

increases from ~6 L/min at rest to >200 L/min in elite endurance athletes, and there is a shift from nasal to mouth breathing. As a consequence, the need to heat and humidify the inhaled air is increased, and abnormal heat and water losses occur within the lower airways. The thermal and osmotic stresses generated by this loss trigger a wide range of vascular, cellular, and neural events, ultimately leading, in susceptible individuals, to airway narrowing. At times of increased ventilatory flow, the mechanical load applied to the airways is increased, and this event could promote airway epithelial injury. Complex interactions between genetic and environmental factors (eg, air pollutants, allergens, and viruses) are likely to modulate the extent of the injury. The consequences of a disrupted airway epithelium are, in the short-term, to facilitate the passage of noxious substances across the airway wall; in the long-term (through repetitive and/or aberrant injury-repair), the possible development of airway hyperresponsiveness (AHR) and tissue remodeling. While there is a theoretical base for the involvement of parasympathetic and neurogenic factors in EIB, human-based evidence is still lacking to confirm the contribution of the nervous system to the pathogenesis of EIB.

EIB OR EXERCISE-INDUCED ASTHMA?

EIB is identified as a transient reduction in lung function after exercise in individuals with or without clinically recognized asthma. A 10% or more decrease in forced expiratory volume in 1 second (FEV_1) after strenuous exercise is widely accepted as evidence for EIB.[2] The term exercise-induced asthma (EIA) describes the same functional change in those with a prior diagnosis of asthma. Both EIB and EIA are typically associated with respiratory symptoms. Yet occurrence of symptoms is not systematic and should not be relied upon for diagnosis.[3,4] The generic term EIB will be used in this article.

The prevalence of EIB is usually estimated around 30% to 50% among individuals with asthma. While EIB is often just one of the many manifestations of asthma, the severity of asthma seems to act as a contributing factor. In a study performed on 164 children with asthma, the prevalence of EIB was greater in those children with moderate or severe persistent asthma (as defined by the Global Initiative for Asthma guidelines) compared with those with intermittent asthma.[5] EIB in childhood has also been suggested as predictor for subsequent development of asthma.[6] However, studies that have assessed EIB in childhood as a risk factor for asthma symptoms in early adulthood have so far produced variable outcomes.[6–9]

Alongside children,[5,10] populations of regular exercisers, such as elite athletes[11] and active-duty military recruits,[12] seem particularly at risk for EIB. In Olympic athletes, EIB has been identified as the most common chronic medical condition, with a prevalence rate of ~8%.[13] While regular exercisers often report the same symptoms as asthmatic individuals on exertion (ie, breathlessness, mucus production, wheezing, cough, and chest tightness),[14] exercise is typically the unique trigger for the airway narrowing and respiratory symptoms in these individuals; therefore EIB is the preferred terminology.

ROLE OF THERMAL STRESS IN EIB

During strenuous exercise, the heating of large volumes of unconditioned air to body temperature is associated with a reduction in the temperature of both the intrathoracic and intrapulmonary airways.[15] Originally, airway cooling was proposed as the stimulus to EIB.[16] This proposal was extended in 1986 to encompass the bronchial vasculature and became known as the thermal theory of EIB.[17] It was proposed that the cooling effect of exercise hyperpnoea causes vasoconstriction of the bronchial circulation. As the exercise ceases and ventilation returns to normal, a reactive hyperemia occurs, leading to vascular leakage and edema formation. The thermal theory proposed that it was the vascular engorgement and edema in the mucosa and submucosa that accounted for the transient airway narrowing of EIB.[18]

Some studies,[17] but not all,[19] have shown that the fall in FEV_1 that followed a short period of hyperpnoea was directly linked to the rate of change in ventilation after the challenge and to the thermal gradient after challenge. Further, a reduction in mucosal blood supply induced by inhalation of norepinephrine was accompanied by limited airway rewarming and by an attenuated airway response.[20]

While thermal stress is likely to contribute to EIB in low temperature conditions, thermal stress is not a prerequisite for EIB. For example, severe EIB has been shown to occur when hot dry air is inspired.[21–24] Moreover cooling the inspired air, while keeping water loss the same, did not necessarily enhance severity of EIB.[25] When the air inspired during exercise is cold, both the thermal and osmotic stresses are likely to be important; first, because inspiring cold air increases the surface area that becomes dehydrated and hyperosmotic, and second because vascular engorgement could amplify the airway narrowing effect of smooth muscle contraction.[26] These events may account for the increased severity of EIB observed in athletes when exercising in the cold.[27,28]

OSMOTIC STRESS AS A PREREQUISITE FOR EIB

The osmotic theory was developed as a consequence of the observations of severe EIB with hot dry air inspirate.[21–23,26] It was proposed that the airway surface liquid (ASL) volume was so small (<1 mL in the first 12 generations of airways) that the evaporative loss in humidifying the air during exercise led to a transient dehydration and increase in ASL osmolarity.[29,30]

According to the mathematical model developed by Daviskas and colleagues,[31] with air of temperate conditions and ventilatory flows of 60 L/min, generations 8 to 10 are recruited in the conditioning process, and a significant amount of water is lost within these small airways (**Fig. 1**). During real-life exercise, individuals often reach ventilatory flows >60 L/min^{-1}, and environmental conditions (such as cold dry air) can exacerbate water loss within the airways. In those situations, even the very small airways (generations 10–12) could be subject to dehydration.

The osmotic theory of EIB proposes that the dehydration of the ASL triggers a cascade of events that involves sequentially: a rise in the osmolarity of the ASL; initial water movement from the surrounding cells toward the airway lumen to rapidly restore the ASL (**Fig. 2**); then the shrinkage of subepithelial cells; release of bronchoconstrictive inflammatory mediators (eg, leukotrienes, prostaglandins, or histamine) during regulatory volume increase; and, in the presence of hyperresponsive airway, bronchial smooth muscle contraction (**Fig. 3**). It is the loss of water from the airway surface and its consequences that is common to both theories, but only the osmotic theory encompasses the release of mediators.

A large body of evidence supports the osmotic theory.[26] The severity of EIB was linked to the water content of inspired air[32] and to the measured water loss at the mouth.[29] The airway response to exercise was significantly blunted in asthmatics when air preconditioned to body temperature and fully saturated with water vapor was inspired.[29,32] The mast-cell stabilizing agents nedocromil sodium and sodium cromoglycate are known to inhibit the obstruction that follows exercise[33] and hyperpnoea of dry air.[34,35] Inhalation of the osmotic agent mannitol can mimic the effects of exercise

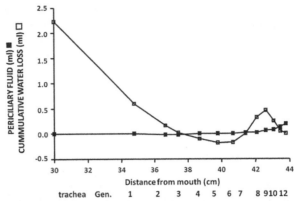

Fig. 1. Cumulative loss of water predicted for each generation from the model of Daviskas[31] under inspiratory conditions of approximately 26°C with 8.8 μL H_2O/L of air (36.5% relative humidity) and for a rate of ventilation of 60 L/min sustained over 8 minutes. The periciliary fluid volume available is also illustrated. The volume of water lost in 8 minutes exceeded the volume of periciliary fluid available in most generations. (*Data from* Anderson SD, Daviskas E, Smith CM. Exercise-induced asthma: a difference in opinion regarding the stimulus. Allergy Proc 1989;10:222.)

on the airway caliber[36,37] and the inflammatory mediator release in asthmatics.[38,39] Athletes in whom dehydration of their airways is more likely to occur (ie, endurance-trained athletes and winter athletes) are at increased risk for EIB.[11]

Recently, it has been suggested that impairment in bronchial airway surface secretions could contribute to dehydration of the ASL during exercise in patients with asthma and in athletes. Using sputum percent solids as a marker for airway hydration, Loughlin and colleagues reported that airway hydration is significantly reduced at baseline in clinically stable asthmatics.[40] Further, athletes with excessive bronchial reactivity have been found to have a reduced ability to sweat.[41] Since respiratory gland epithelium and sweat gland epithelium share identical mechanisms of muscarinic receptor (m3 subtype)-dependent sodium, chloride, and water secretion, this latest result may indicate a general deficiency in body fluid homeostasis regulation in those individuals with EIB. From a mechanical viewpoint, mice deficient with aquaporin 5, a water channel protein expressed in alveolar type 1 cells of the lungs, appear hyper-reactive to bronchoconstriction.[42] Further studies are required to confirm the role of aquaporin 5 in the pathogenesis of EIB in humans.

EPITHELIAL DISRUPTION AS A CONSEQUENCE OF THE THERMAL STRESS

The volume of ASL is critical for proper lung defense. When the depth of the ASL is reduced, the integrity of the epithelial barrier is compromised, and epithelial cell injury is likely to occur. In animals, hyperventilation of dry air has been shown to cause significant desquamation of the airway epithelium,[43,44] with the extent of injury being dependent upon ventilatory flow and dryness of the air.[45] In asthmatic individuals with EIB, induced sputum samples obtained after exercise revealed significant airway damage, with an increased concentration of columnar epithelial cells that correlated with the release of the inflammatory mediators histamine and leukotrienes.[46] Using the lung-specific protein Clara cell CC16 as an index for airway permeability, the authors[47,48] and others[49,50] confirmed that strenuous exercise transiently compromises the integrity of the airway epithelial barrier.

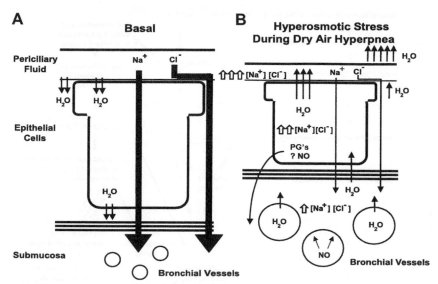

Fig. 2. Epithelial cells and ion transport under basal conditions (*A*) and hyperosmotic stress during dry air hyperpnoea (*B*). Under basal conditions, Na$^+$ ions are absorbed via an apical sodium channel, and Cl$^-$ ions move paracellularly. Under basal conditions, water moves into the epithelial cells and submucosa due to the osmotic gradient created by the movement of these ions. During hyperpnoea, evaporative water loss reduces the periciary fluid layer and increases the ion concentration, which creates an osmotic stimulus for water to move out of the epithelial cells. As a result, the epithelial cells shrink, creating an osmotic stimulus for water to move from the submucosa. Hyperosmolarity of the epithelial cells and the submucosa is a possible stimulus for the release of nitric oxide (NO) and prostaglandins (PGs). These substances may contribute to the increase in the blood flow documented in people breathing dry air. (*From* Anderson SD, Daviskas E. Airway drying and exercise-induced asthma. In: McFadden ER, editor. Exercise-induced asthma—lung biology in health and disease. New York: Marcel Dekker; 1999. p. 91; with permission.)

In the short term, breaches in the airway epithelial barrier could, among other events, transiently facilitate the passage of inhaled substances (ie, viruses, bacteria, allergens, or airborne pollutants or irritants) across the airway epithelium and increase the interaction of those substances with resident immune and inflammatory cells, trigger an inflammatory response with consequent infiltration of mast cells[51] and secondary influx of neutrophils,[49] cause the loss of the bronchoprotective agent prostaglandin E$_2$,[46,52] and impede mucociliary clearance.[53] Either alone or in combination, these factors could initiate acute airway narrowing following exercise.

DOES MECHANICAL STRESS CONTRIBUTE TO AIRWAY INJURY?

Although dehydration stress is regarded as the most important precursor of airway epithelial injury during exercise, the role of mechanical stress cannot be excluded.

During respiration, the airways are subjected to complex physical forces. Movement of air across the surface of the airway imparts a shear stress on the surface epithelium. Mathematical modeling has shown that at a peak flow rate of 1 L/s (representing normal expiratory flow), wall shear stress in the major airways reaches up to 0.9 Pa.[54] At 8 L/s (representing cough), the maximum value for wall shear stress rises to 19 Pa.[54] Cough, through wall shear stresses, is thought to be a contributing factor to

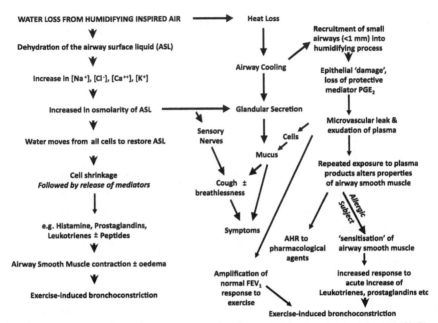

Fig. 3. Flow chart describing the acute events leading to EIB in the classic asthmatic (*left*) and the events leading to the development of EIB in the athlete (*right*). (*From* Anderson SD, Kippelen P. Exercise-induced bronchoconstriction: pathogenesis. Curr Allergy Asthma Rep 2005;5:117; with permission.)

airway injury, inflammation, and obstruction.[55] During exercise, the increased osmolarity of the ASL is likely to activate sensory nerves and trigger cough.[56] Cough on exertion is often considered as a clinical manifestation of asthma. Moreover, cough is commonly reported by elite athletes,[57] especially during the winter months.[58] Hyperpnoea of cold air is known to stimulate cough.[59] Cough, through wall shear stresses, may therefore contribute to the high prevalence of AHR, inflammation, and remodeling in cold-weather athletes.[60,61]

During exercise, stretching of the airway wall and steeper transairway pressure gradients could cause deformation of the epithelial cells. Mechanical deformation of epithelial cells is accompanied by signaling, structural, and mechanical responses[62] that may impact on airway function and cause additional trauma to an already inflamed epithelial layer. However, high physical forces are not all bad for the airways. Deep breaths, as occurs spontaneously with exercise, are regarded as among the most potent bronchodilator agents.[63] In healthy individuals, deep breaths are thought to help to maintain airway patency through disruption of the force-generating machinery (ie, detachment of cross bridges). In asthmatics, however, the bronchodilator effect of tidal breathing muscle stretches is often lost.[64] As a consequence, the onset of EIB may sometimes occur during exercise in patients with asthma.[65,66]

EPITHELIAL INJURY IN THE DEVELOPMENT OF EIB

In the long term, interaction between a disrupted airway epithelium and environmental stimuli could lead to functional and structural changes within the airways.

To restore the integrity of the airway epithelial barrier and maintain homeostasis, injury is rapidly followed by repair. The injury–repair processes are known to produce, by themselves, a series of physiologic and cellular events within the airways that promote inflammation and tissue repair. An immediate response to the denudation of the airway epithelium in vivo is plasma exudation.[67] Strong secretory and exudative responses ensure that a gel-like network of fibrin and other attached proteins covers the denuded basement membrane, which then helps to maintain mucosal defense and assist in the restoration process.[67] In parallel, de-differentiation and migration of basal and Clara cells ensure a rapid restoration of the epithelium.[68] Rapid and well-orchestrated injury–repair processes are critical in ensuring that the airway epithelium keeps protecting the internal milieu from external noxious agents.

During exercise hyperpnoea, the exposure of the airways to environmental stimuli is increased. In the presence of environmental triggers and with a susceptible airway epithelium (such as in asthma), not only does penetration of external noxious agents increase, but aberrant repair may also occur. A defect in epithelial tight junctions has recently been observed in patients with asthma.[69] Moreover, an in vitro study has implicated a decreased production of fibronectin (ie, 1 of the primary extracellular matrix proteins) in dysregulated repair of asthmatic epithelium.[70] A dysregulated (or aberrant) repair may lead, among other things, to the generation of growth factors and to an ineffective resolution of inflammation (with increased cytotoxicity).[71] Through interaction with the underlying mesenchyme, growth factors and cytokines could then promote tissue remodeling and persistent inflammation (**Fig. 4**). In asthma with EIB, airway epithelial injury has been observed at rest,[52] and exercise has been shown to exacerbate the degree of airway injury.[46]

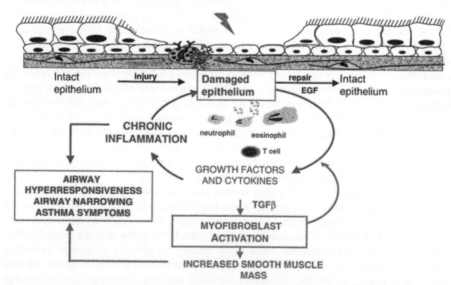

Fig. 4. Model for the interaction between environmental agents and a susceptible epithelium as a trigger for persistent airway inflammation and remodeling in asthma. Susceptibility to environmental oxidants causes epithelial damage, which triggers a normal injury–repair response involving release of mediators that promote inflammation and tissue repair (which involves transient remodeling responses). However, the release of endogenous oxidants by inflammatory cells causes further injury to the susceptible epithelium, resulting in a chronic state of tissue damage, which maintains the appropriate environment for persistent inflammation and tissue remodeling. (*From* Davies DE, Holgate ST. Asthma: the importance of epithelial mesenchymal communication in pathogenesis. Inflammation and the airway epithelium in asthma. Int J Biochem Cell Biol 2002;34:1524; with permission.)

In a susceptible airway epithelium, the inflammatory cell influx that follows tissue injury may also initiate secondary damage through production of endogenous reactive oxygen.[71] In asthmatic children and adolescents with EIB levels of 8-isoprostane in exhaled breath condensate are increased.[72] Moreover, an increase in the body's anti-oxidant capacity through supplementation with undenatured whey protein[73] or ascorbic acid[74] has been shown to significantly reduce the severity of EIB.

In nonasthmatic individuals whose airways are repetitively exposed to injury (such as elite athletes), rather than aberrant repair, it is the high frequency of the injury–repair process that could favor the development of EIB. In this population, transient but repeated leakage of bulk plasma could, via chronic exposure of the airway smooth muscle to biologically active molecules (eg, growth factors and cytokines), modify the contractile properties of the muscle, rendering it hyper-responsive (see **Fig. 3**). High prevalence of AHR has been observed in many elite athletes, particularly in those sustaining high ventilatory flows (ie, endurance-trained athletes) or those exposed to cold dry air (ie, winter athletes) or to noxious environmental conditions (eg, swim-mers).[11,75–77] Moreover, atopy is a strong risk factor for EIB in elite athletes.[78] In athletes with allergies, repeated injury–repair could create a model of passive sensiti-zation,[79] whereby the smooth muscle would be repetitively exposed to circulating immunoglublin E (IgE) and would promote the development of EIB (see **Fig. 3**).

CONTRIBUTION OF THE NERVOUS SYSTEM IN EIB

Parasympathetic innervation of the human airways regulates many aspects of airway function, including bronchial smooth muscle contraction, mucus secretion, and vaso-dilatation of the bronchial vasculature, all of which are involved in EIB. Through acti-vation of muscarinic receptors present on extraneuronal cells, such as epithelial cells and inflammatory cells,[80] parasympathetic signaling may also contribute to airway inflammation and tissue remodeling.[81,82] Thus far, however, the evidence for the involvement of the cholinergic system in EIB, via the use of the inhaled anticholin-ergic agent ipratropium bromide, has been conflicting.[83–86] Moreover, the therapeutic effect of ipratropium on EIB seems to vary greatly among individuals.[87] This high vari-ability has been attributed to interindividual differences in vagal activity.[88] Vagal activ-ity is known to increase in endurance-trained athletes,[89] and endurance athletes are particularly prone to EIB.[11] Therefore it cannot be excluded that, in regular exercisers, the cholinergic system contributes to the development EIB.[90]

Both chemical agents and physical factors (such as mechanical probing, dry gas hyperpnoea, and hypertonic aerosols) have the potential to activate sensory nerves endings from bronchopulmonary C-fibers and trigger the release of sensory neuro-peptides (eg, substance P, neurokinin A, and calcitonin gene-related peptide).[91] In animals, sensory neuropeptides have been shown to directly modulate bronchial tone, bronchovascular caliber and permeability, and secretions.[91] These effects seem mainly mediated by the interaction between sensory neuropeptides substance P and neurokinin A with tachykinin (NK_1, NK_2) receptors, as demonstrated in patients with asthma.[92] However, thus far, limited human-based evidence supports the role of sensory neuropeptides in EIB. The inhalation of the selective NK_1 receptor antagonist FK-888 before exercise in asthmatic patients did not inhibit EIB.[93] However, the recov-ery from EIB was somewhat accelerated with FK-888, which led the authors to postu-late that NK_1 receptor-mediated mechanisms are involved in the recovery phase of EIB.

A novel theory is that, in asthmatic individuals, bronchoconstriction and mucus release after exercise could be partly mediated by retrograde axonal transmission via neurokinin A release.[94] The theory proposes that, in the presence of an osmotic stress (such as during exercise), the disrupted airway epithelium of asthmatic patients with EIB causes sustained production of inflammatory eicosonoids, particularly cysteinyl–leukotrienes (cys-LTs). Cyst-LTs then activate sensory nerves containing neurokinins, which, in turn, initiate contraction of the bronchial smooth muscle and release of mucin. Significant release of de novo synthesized eicosanoids has been noticed in vitro following osmotic challenge of human mast cells.[95] Moreover, production of cys-LTs is known to be increased in asthmatic patients with EIB.[52,96] Recently, in asthmatic patients with EIB, exercise was associated with increased release of goblet cell mucin 5AC (MUC5AC) and of cyst-LTs into the airways.[97] In the same study, levels of cyst-LTs in induced sputum were positively correlated with levels of neurokinin A.[97] Altogether, these results support the idea that neurokinin A release through sensory nerve activation may partly mediate contraction of the airway smooth muscle and overproduction of mucus in EIB.

SUMMARY

EIB occurs in individuals with and without clinically recognized asthma. EIB is a functional consequence of the overwhelming of the humidifying process of the airways during exercise. Loss of water associated with exercise hyperpnoea leads to a rise in the osmolarity of the ASL, which causes inflammatory cells to release mediators of bronchoconstriction. During exercise in the cold, the loss of heat associated with hyperpnoea may lead to vascular engorgement as the airways rewarm after exercise and may precipitate or enhance airway narrowing. The multiple stressors (ie, heat, osmotic and mechanical stress) to which the airway wall is exposed during exercise are thought to cause injury to the airway epithelium and to trigger an injury–repair cascade. In individuals with a particular genetic make-up (eg, asthmatic individuals), aberrant repair of the airway epithelium could promote airway remodeling responses and a chronic and persistent inflammatory response, leading to EIB development/progression. In regular exercisers, it is the repetitive nature of the injury–repair processes that is thought, via release of bioactive substances, to change the contractile properties of the smooth muscle and induce AHR and promote EIB. Strategies to provide protection to the airways against environmental insults and/or to enhance the ability of the epithelium to withstand stresses during exercise should be devised to limit development/progression of the disease.

REFERENCES

1. Becker JM, Rogers J, Rossini G, et al. Asthma deaths during sports: report of a 7-year experience. J Allergy Clin Immunol 2004;113:264–7.
2. Crapo RO, Casaburi R, Coates AL, et al. Guidelines for methacholine and exercise challenge testing-1999. This official statement of the American Thoracic Society was adopted by the ATS Board of Directors, July 1999. Am J Respir Crit Care Med 2000;161:309–29.
3. Rundell KW, Im J, Mayers LB, et al. Self-reported symptoms and exercise-induced asthma in the elite athlete. Med Sci Sports Exerc 2001;33:208–13.
4. De Baets F, Bodart E, Dramaix-Wilmet M, et al. Exercise-induced respiratory symptoms are poor predictors of bronchoconstriction. Pediatr Pulmonol 2005; 39:301–5.
5. Cabral AL, Conceição GM, Fonseca-Guedes CH, et al. Exercise-induced bronchospasm in children: effects of asthma severity. Am J Respir Crit Care Med 1999;159:1819–23.

6. Porsbjerg C, von Linstow ML, Ulrik CS, et al. Outcome in adulthood of asymptomatic airway hyperresponsiveness to histamine and exercise-induced bronchospasm in childhood. Ann Allergy Asthma Immunol 2005;95:137–42.

7. Riiser A, Hovland V, Carlsen KH, et al. Does bronchial hyperresponsiveness in childhood predict active asthma in adolescence? Am J Respir Crit Care Med 2012;186:493–500.

8. Rasmussen F, Lambrechtsen J, Siersted HC, et al. Asymptomatic bronchial hyperresponsiveness to exercise in childhood and the development of asthma related symptoms in young adulthood: the Odense Schoolchild Study. Thorax 1999;54:587–9.

9. Jones A. Asymptomatic bronchial hyperreactivity and the development of asthma and other respiratory tract illnesses in children. Thorax 1994;49:757–61.

10. Benarab-Boucherit Y, Mehdioui H, Nedjar F, et al. Prevalence rate of exercise-induced bronchoconstriction in Annaba (Algeria) schoolchildren. J Asthma 2011;48:511–6.

11. Carlsen KH, Anderson SD, Bjermer L, et al. Exercise-induced asthma, respiratory and allergic disorders in elite athletes: epidemiology, mechanisms and diagnosis: part I of the report from the Joint Task Force of the European Respiratory Society (ERS) and the European Academy of Allergy and Clinical Immunology (EAACI) in cooperation with GA2LEN. Allergy 2008;63:387–403.

12. Holley AB, Cohee B, Walter RJ, et al. Eucapnic voluntary hyperventilation is superior to methacholine challenge testing for detecting airway hyperreactivity in non-athletes. J Asthma 2012;49:614–9.

13. Fitch KD. An overview of asthma and airway hyper-responsiveness in Olympic athletes. Br J Sports Med 2012;46(6):413–6.

14. Turcotte H, Langdeau JB, Thibault G, et al. Prevalence of respiratory symptoms in an athlete population. Respir Med 2003;97:955–63.

15. McFadden ER, Pichurko BM, Bowman HF, et al. Thermal mapping of the airways in humans. J Appl Physiol 1985;58:564–70.

16. Deal EC, McFadden ER, Ingram RH, et al. Role of respiratory heat exchange in production of exercise-induced asthma. J Appl Physiol 1979;46:467–75.

17. McFadden ER, Lenner KA, Strohl KP. Postexertional airway rewarming and thermally induced asthma. New insights into pathophysiology and possible pathogenesis. J Clin Invest 1986;78:18–25.

18. McFadden ER. Hypothesis: exercise-induced asthma as a vascular phenomenon. Lancet 1990;335:880–3.

19. Smith CM, Anderson SD, Walsh S, et al. An investigation of the effects of heat and water exchange in the recovery period after exercise in children with asthma. Am Rev Respir Dis 1989;140:598–605.

20. Gilbert IA, McFadden ER. Airway cooling and rewarming. The second reaction sequence in exercise-induced asthma. J Clin Invest 1992;90:699–704.

21. Anderson SD, Schoeffel RE, Black JL, et al. Airway cooling as the stimulus to exercise-induced asthma—a re-evaluation. Eur J Respir Dis 1985;67:20–30.

22. Anderson SD, Daviskas E. The airway microvasculature and exercise induced asthma. Thorax 1992;47:748–52.

23. Eschenbacher WL, Moore TB, Lorenzen TJ, et al. Pulmonary responses of asthmatic and normal subjects to different temperature and humidity conditions in an environmental chamber. Lung 1992;170:51–62.

24. Aitken ML, Marini JJ. Effect of heat delivery and extraction on airway conductance in normal and in asthmatic subjects. Am Rev Respir Dis 1985;131:357–61.

25. Hahn A, Anderson SD, Morton AR, et al. A reinterpretation of the effect of temperature and water content of the inspired air in exercise-induced asthma. Am Rev Respir Dis 1984;130:575–9.
26. Anderson SD, Daviskas E. The mechanism of exercise-induced asthma is…. J Allergy Clin Immunol 2000;106:453–9.
27. Stensrud T, Berntsen S, Carlsen KH. Exercise capacity and exercise-induced bronchoconstriction (EIB) in a cold environment. Respir Med 2007;101:1529–36.
28. Anderson SD, Holzer K. Exercise-induced asthma: is it the right diagnosis in elite athletes? J Allergy Clin Immunol 2000;106:419–28.
29. Anderson SD, Schoeffel RE, Follet R, et al. Sensitivity to heat and water loss at rest and during exercise in asthmatic patients. Eur J Respir Dis 1982;63:459–71.
30. Anderson SD. Is there a unifying hypothesis for exercise-induced asthma? J Allergy Clin Immunol 1984;73:660–5.
31. Daviskas E, Gonda I, Anderson SD. Local airway heat and water vapour losses. Respir Physiol 1991;84:115–32.
32. Strauss RH, McFadden ER, Ingram RH, et al. Influence of heat and humidity on the airway obstruction induced by exercise in asthma. J Clin Invest 1978;61:433–40.
33. Spooner CH, Spooner GR, Rowe BH. Mast-cell stabilising agents to prevent exercise-induced bronchoconstriction. Cochrane Database Syst Rev 2003;(4):CD002307.
34. Pfleger A, Eber E, Weinhandl E, et al. Effects of nedocromil and salbutamol on airway reactivity in children with asthma. Eur Respir J 2002;20:624–9.
35. Kippelen P, Larsson J, Anderson SD, et al. Effect of sodium cromoglycate on mast cell mediators during hyperpnea in athletes. Med Sci Sports Exerc 2010;42:1853–60.
36. Brannan JD, Koskela H, Anderson SD, et al. Responsiveness to mannitol in asthmatic subjects with exercise- and hyperventilation-induced asthma. Am J Respir Crit Care Med 1998;158:1120–6.
37. Barben J, Kuehni CE, Strippoli MP, et al. Mannitol dry powder challenge in comparison with exercise testing in children. Pediatr Pulmonol 2011;46:842–8.
38. Brannan JD, Gulliksson M, Anderson SD, et al. Evidence of mast cell activation and leukotriene release after mannitol inhalation. Eur Respir J 2003;22:491–6.
39. Brannan JD, Gulliksson M, Anderson SD, et al. Inhibition of mast cell PGD2 release protects against mannitol-induced airway narrowing. Eur Respir J 2006;27:944–50.
40. Loughlin CE, Esther CR, Lazarowski ER, et al. Neutrophilic inflammation is associated with altered airway hydration in stable asthmatics. Respir Med 2010;104:29–33.
41. Park C, Stafford C, Lockette W. Exercise-induced asthma may be associated with diminished sweat secretion rates in humans. Chest 2008;134:552–8.
42. Krane CM, Fortner CN, Hand AR, et al. Aquaporin 5-deficient mouse lungs are hyperresponsive to cholinergic stimulation. Proc Natl Acad Sci U S A 2001;98:14114–9.
43. Omori C, Schofield BH, Mitzner W, et al. Hyperpnea with dry air causes time-dependent alterations in mucosal morphology and bronchovascular permeability. J Appl Physiol 1995;78:1043–51.
44. Barbet JP, Chauveau M, Labbé S, et al. Breathing dry air causes acute epithelial damage and inflammation of the guinea pig trachea. J Appl Physiol 1988;64:1851–7.

45. Freed AN, Omori C, Schofield BH, et al. Dry air-induced mucosal cell injury and bronchovascular leakage in canine peripheral airways. Am J Respir Cell Mol Biol 1994;11:724–32.

46. Hallstrand TS, Moody MW, Wurfel MM, et al. Inflammatory basis of exercise-induced bronchoconstriction. Am J Respir Crit Care Med 2005;172:679–86.

47. Bolger C, Tufvesson E, Anderson SD, et al. The effect of inspired air conditions on exercise-induced bronchoconstriction and urinary CC16 levels in athletes. J Appl Physiol 2011;111(4):1059–65.

48. Bolger C, Tufvesson E, Sue-Chu M, et al. Hyperpnea-induced bronchoconstriction and urinary CC16 levels in athletes. Med Sci Sports Exerc 2011;43:1207–13.

49. Chimenti L, Morici G, Paternò A, et al. Bronchial epithelial damage after a half-marathon in nonasthmatic amateur runners. Am J Physiol Lung Cell Mol Physiol 2010;298:L857–62.

50. Romberg K, Bjermer L, Tufvesson E. Exercise but not mannitol provocation increases urinary Clara cell protein (CC16) in elite swimmers. Respir Med 2011;105:31–6.

51. Davis MS, Schofield B, Freed AN. Repeated peripheral airway hyperpnea causes inflammation and remodeling in dogs. Med Sci Sports Exerc 2003;35:608–16.

52. Hallstrand TS, Moody MW, Aitken ML, et al. Airway immunopathology of asthma with exercise-induced bronchoconstriction. J Allergy Clin Immunol 2005;116:586–93.

53. Daviskas E, Anderson SD, Gonda I, et al. Changes in mucociliary clearance during and after isocapnic hyperventilation in asthmatic and healthy subjects. Eur Respir J 1995;8:742–51.

54. Green AS. Modeling of peak-flow wall shear stress in major airways of the lung. J Biomech 2004;37:661–7.

55. Chowdhary R, Singh V, Tattersfield AE, et al. Relationship of flow and cross-sectional area to frictional stress in airway models of asthma. J Asthma 1999; 36:419–26.

56. Anderson SD, Kippelen P. Exercise-induced bronchoconstriction: pathogenesis. Curr Allergy Asthma Rep 2005;5:116–22.

57. Boulet LP. Cough and upper airway disorders in elite athletes: a critical review. Br J Sports Med 2012;46(6):417–21.

58. Turmel J, Bougault V, Boulet LP. Seasonal variations of cough reflex sensitivity in elite athletes training in cold air environment. Cough 2012;8:2.

59. Banner AS, Chausow A, Green J. The tussive effect of hyperpnea with cold air. Am Rev Respir Dis 1985;131:362–7.

60. Karjalainen EM, Laitinen A, Sue-Chu M, et al. Evidence of airway inflammation and remodeling in ski athletes with and without bronchial hyperresponsiveness to methacholine. Am J Respir Crit Care Med 2000;161:2086–91.

61. Sue-Chu M, Larsson L, Moen T, et al. Bronchoscopy and bronchoalveolar lavage findings in cross-country skiers with and without "ski asthma". Eur Respir J 1999; 13:626–32.

62. Tschumperlin DJ, Drazen JM. Chronic effects of mechanical force on airways. Annu Rev Physiol 2006;68:563–83.

63. Gump A, Haughney L, Fredberg J. Relaxation of activated airway smooth muscle: relative potency of isoproterenol vs. tidal stretch. J Appl Physiol 2001;90:2306–10.

64. Jensen A, Atileh H, Suki B, et al. Selected contribution: airway caliber in healthy and asthmatic subjects: effects of bronchial challenge and deep inspirations. J Appl Physiol 2001;91:506–15 [discussion: 504–5].

65. Suman OE, Babcock MA, Pegelow DF, et al. Airway obstruction during exercise in asthma. Am J Respir Crit Care Med 1995;152:24–31.

66. van Leeuwen JC, Driessen JM, de Jongh FH, et al. Monitoring pulmonary function during exercise in children with asthma. Arch Dis Child 2011;96:664–8.
67. Erjefält JS, Erjefält I, Sundler F, et al. Microcirculation-derived factors in airway epithelial repair in vivo. Microvasc Res 1994;48:161–78.
68. Erjefält JS, Erjefält I, Sundler F, et al. In vivo restitution of airway epithelium. Cell Tissue Res 1995;281:305–16.
69. Xiao C, Puddicombe SM, Field S, et al. Defective epithelial barrier function in asthma. J Allergy Clin Immunol 2011;128:549–556.e1–12.
70. Kicic A, Hallstrand TS, Sutanto EN, et al. Decreased fibronectin production significantly contributes to dysregulated repair of asthmatic epithelium. Am J Respir Crit Care Med 2010;181:889–98.
71. Holgate ST. Epithelium dysfunction in asthma. J Allergy Clin Immunol 2007;120: 1233–44 [quiz: 1245–6].
72. Barreto M, Villa MP, Olita C, et al. 8-Isoprostane in exhaled breath condensate and exercise-induced bronchoconstriction in asthmatic children and adolescents. Chest 2009;135:66–73.
73. Baumann JM, Rundell KW, Evans TM, et al. Effects of cysteine donor supplementation on exercise-induced bronchoconstriction. Med Sci Sports Exerc 2005;37: 1468–73.
74. Tecklenburg SL, Mickleborough TD, Fly AD, et al. Ascorbic acid supplementation attenuates exercise-induced bronchoconstriction in patients with asthma. Respir Med 2007;101:1770–8.
75. Bougault V, Turmel J, St-Laurent J, et al. Asthma, airway inflammation, and epithelial damage in swimmers and cold-air athletes. Eur Respir J 2009;33:740–6.
76. Sue-Chu M, Brannan JD, Anderson SD, et al. Airway hyperresponsiveness to methacholine, adenosine 5-monophosphate, mannitol, eucapnic voluntary hyperpnoea and field exercise challenge in elite cross-country skiers. Br J Sports Med 2010;44:827–32.
77. Helenius IJ, Tikkanen HO, Haahtela T. Occurrence of exercise-induced bronchospasm in elite runners: dependence on atopy and exposure to cold air and pollen. Br J Sports Med 1998;32:125–9.
78. Helenius IJ, Tikkanen HO, Sarna S, et al. Asthma and increased bronchial responsiveness in elite athletes: atopy and sport event as risk factors. J Allergy Clin Immunol 1998;101:646–52.
79. Anderson SD, Kippelen P. Airway injury as a mechanism for exercise-induced bronchoconstriction in elite athletes. J Allergy Clin Immunol 2008;122:225–35 [quiz: 236–7].
80. Wessler I, Kirkpatrick CJ. Acetylcholine beyond neurons: the non-neuronal cholinergic system in humans. Br J Pharmacol 2008;154:1558–71.
81. Oenema TA, Kolahian S, Nanninga JE, et al. Pro-inflammatory mechanisms of muscarinic receptor stimulation in airway smooth muscle. Respir Res 2010; 11:130.
82. Gosens R, Bos IS, Zaagsma J, et al. Protective effects of tiotropium bromide in the progression of airway smooth muscle remodeling. Am J Respir Crit Care Med 2005;171:1096–102.
83. Poppius H, Sovijärvi AR, Tammilehto L. Lack of protective effect of high-dose ipratropium on bronchoconstriction following exercise with cold air breathing in patients with mild asthma. Eur J Respir Dis 1986;68:319–25.
84. Borut TC, Tashkin DP, Fischer TJ, et al. Comparison of aerosolized atropine sulfate and SCH 1000 on exercise-induced bronchospasm in children. J Allergy Clin Immunol 1977;60:127–33.

85. Boulet LP, Turcotte H, Tennina S. Comparative efficacy of salbutamol, ipratropium, and cromoglycate in the prevention of bronchospasm induced by exercise and hyperosmolar challenges. J Allergy Clin Immunol 1989;83:882–7.
86. Boaventura LC, Araujo AC, Martinez JB, et al. Effects of ipratropium on exercise-induced bronchospasm. Int J Sports Med 2010;31:516–20.
87. Boner AL, Vallone G, De Stefano G. Effect of inhaled ipratropium bromide on methacholine and exercise provocation in asthmatic children. Pediatr Pulmonol 1989;6:81–5.
88. Knöpfli BH, Bar-Or O, Araújo CG. Effect of ipratropium bromide on EIB in children depends on vagal activity. Med Sci Sports Exerc 2005;37:354–9.
89. Goldsmith RL, Bigger JT, Steinman RC, et al. Comparison of 24-hour parasympathetic activity in endurance-trained and untrained young men. J Am Coll Cardiol 1992;20:552–8.
90. Langdeau JB, Turcotte H, Desagné P, et al. Influence of sympatho-vagal balance on airway responsiveness in athletes. Eur J Appl Physiol 2000;83:370–5.
91. Solway J, Leff AR. Sensory neuropeptides and airway function. J Appl Physiol 1991;71:2077–87.
92. Joos GF, Vincken W, Louis R, et al. Dual tachykinin NK1/NK2 antagonist DNK333 inhibits neurokinin A-induced bronchoconstriction in asthma patients. Eur Respir J 2004;23:76–81.
93. Ichinose M, Miura M, Yamauchi H, et al. A neurokinin 1-receptor antagonist improves exercise-induced airway narrowing in asthmatic patients. Am J Respir Crit Care Med 1996;153:936–41.
94. Hallstrand TS. New insights into pathogenesis of exercise-induced bronchoconstriction. Curr Opin Allergy Clin Immunol 2012;12:42–8.
95. Gulliksson M, Palmberg L, Nilsson G, et al. Release of prostaglandin D2 and leukotriene C4 in response to hyperosmolar stimulation of mast cells. Allergy 2006;61:1473–9.
96. Carraro S, Corradi M, Zanconato S, et al. Exhaled breath condensate cysteinyl leukotrienes are increased in children with exercise-induced bronchoconstriction. J Allergy Clin Immunol 2005;115:764–70.
97. Hallstrand TS, Debley JS, Farin FM, et al. Role of MUC5AC in the pathogenesis of exercise-induced bronchoconstriction. J Allergy Clin Immunol 2007;119:1092–8.

Role of Cells and Mediators in Exercise-Induced Bronchoconstriction

Teal S. Hallstrand, MD, MPH[a],*, William A. Altemeier, MD[a],
Moira L. Aitken, MD[a], William R. Henderson Jr, MD[b]

KEYWORDS

- Asthma • Eicosanoid • Eosinophil • Exercise-induced bronchoconstriction
- Leukotriene • Mast cell • Phospholipase • Prostaglandin

KEY POINTS

- Patients who are susceptible to exercise-induced bronchoconstriction have epithelial shedding, infiltration of the airways with mast cells and eosinophils, and increased production of inflammatory mediators such as leukotrienes.
- During exercise and hyperpnea the inspired air is equilibrated to the conditions of the lower airways, resulting in the transfer of water out of the airways.
- Following exercise challenge, mediators such as cysteinyl leukotrienes and prostaglandin D_2 are released into the airways from mast cells and eosinophils.
- Sensory nerves may mediate the effects of cysteinyl leukotrienes and other lipid mediators, leading to smooth-muscle contraction and mucus release.
- The epithelium may serve as a regulator of leukocyte activation in response to water loss or osmotic stress, but the mechanism remains incompletely understood.

INTRODUCTION

The role of inflammatory mediators in the pathogenesis of exercise-induced bronchoconstriction (EIB) has become increasingly clear from studies conducted in human subjects with asthma over the last 15 years. These results indicate very clearly that

Funding: Supported by National Institutes of Health grant HL089215.
Disclosures: T.S. Hallstrand has received research grants from the NIH, American Lung Association, has served as a consultant for Amgen and TEVA pharmaceuticals, and has received lecture fees from Merck & Co. W.R. Henderson has served on advisory boards for Gilead Sciences, has received lecture fees from Merck & Co., and has received industry-sponsored grants from Genentech and Gilead Sciences. W.A. Altemeier and M.L. Aitken have no conflicts of interest.
[a] Division of Pulmonary and Critical Care, Department of Medicine, University of Washington, 1959 NE Pacific Street, Box 356522, Seattle, WA 98195-6522, USA; [b] Division of Allergy and Infectious Diseases, Department of Medicine, UW Medicine at South Lake Union, University of Washington, 850 Republican Street, Seattle, WA 98109-4725, USA
* Corresponding author.
E-mail address: tealh@uw.edu

mediators from mast cells and other airway leukocytes are released into the airways following exercise challenge in individuals who are susceptible to EIB. The evidence that the release of such mediators plays a causal role in the pathogenesis of EIB is strongest for the cysteinyl leukotrienes (CysLTs) C_4, D_4, and E_4, in part because of the availability of receptor antagonists and synthesis inhibitors that alter the leukotriene (LT) pathway. It is also apparent that several other mediators that may play important roles in the pathogenesis of EIB are released into the airways, but the precise roles of these mediators are inferred from animal studies and from the basic biological function of the mediators. Many unanswered questions remain, including why leukocytes become activated in the airways, how either evaporative water loss or the addition of a hyperosmolar solution to the airways initiates downstream cellular effects, and what the connection is between the epithelium and these events that leads to leukocyte activation.

ALTERATIONS IN THE AIRWAYS THAT LEAD TO EIB

As a prototypical feature of indirect airway hyperresponsiveness (AHR), EIB shares common features with other stimuli such as hypertonic aerosols and adenosine, which cause bronchoconstriction through the release of mediators.[1] EIB is only weakly related to structural alterations of the lung[2–4] and airway smooth-muscle hyperresponsiveness measured by direct-acting agonists of smooth-muscle contraction such as methacholine.[5] In one study of 27 asthmatic children, there was no relationship between the methacholine PC_{20} and maximum decrease in forced expiratory volume in 1 second (FEV_1) after exercise ($r = -0.2$, $P = .40$). Another study of elite athletes found that 9 of 25 elite athletes with a positive eucapnic voluntary hyperpnea (EVH) challenge, a surrogate for exercise challenge, had a positive methacholine challenge, demonstrating the discordance between these 2 different features of AHR.[6] Collectively, these studies indicate that EIB is pathophysiologically distinct from other features of asthma, but shares common features with other forms of indirect AHR. A clear understanding of the pathophysiology of EIB is important, as EIB at an early age is associated with the persistence of asthma later in life.[7–9] There is also evidence that chronic lung disease early in life is a risk factor for the development or persistence of EIB later in life.[10]

As subjects with asthma can be characterized based on the presence or absence of EIB using a dry air exercise challenge test, several studies have made comparisons between asthmatics with and without EIB to better understand the basis for EIB. An inflammatory basis of EIB is suggested by an increase in the fraction of exhaled nitric oxide (F_{ENO}) among asthmatics who are susceptible to EIB,[11] especially in subjects with atopy.[12] Although differences in the concentration of inflammatory lipid mediators have not been identified in studies evaluating metabolites in the urine,[13] the concentrations of inflammatory lipid mediators are increased in the airways of individuals with EIB.[2,4,14] In particular, the concentration of CysLTs is increased in induced sputum of adults with EIB,[4] and in exhaled breath condensate (EBC) of children with EIB.[2] In addition, the levels of 8-isoprostanes, nonenzymatic products of phospholipid oxidation, are increased in EBC of asthmatics with EIB, and correlate with the severity of EIB.[14] There is also evidence of a reduction in the formation of protective lipid mediators in the airways such as lipoxin A4 in patients with EIB.[15] Prostaglandin E_2 (PGE_2) is a key regulatory eicosanoid that inhibits EIB when administered by inhalation.[16] The production of PGE_2 relative to CysLTs is reduced in patients with EIB.[4] As the epithelium is a major source of PGE_2, it is notable that the number of epithelial cells shed into the induced sputum is greater in patients with EIB.[4]

The intensity of cellular inflammation in the airways may be an important factor in the susceptibility to EIB, as the formation of inflammatory eicosanoids such as CysLTs and PGD_2 is largely restricted to myeloid cells, especially mast cells that contain leukotriene C_4 (LTC_4) and prostaglandin D_2 (PGD_2) synthases and eosinophils that also contain LTC_4 synthase.[17] Several studies have associated the degree of sputum eosinophilia with the severity of EIB,[4] although sputum eosinophilia is not present in all patients with EIB.[4] A recent study of the effect of inhaled corticosteroid (ICS) cicleso-nide in steroid-naïve asthmatic patients with EIB found that the magnitude and onset of the suppression of EIB in response to high-dose, but not low-dose, ICS therapy was associated with the degree of sputum eosinophilia.[18]

In a genome-wide expression study of airway cells, the authors identified a unique molecular phenotype of EIB-positive asthmatics relative to asthmatic individuals without EIB, notable for the increased expression of mast cell, mucus, and epithelial repair genes.[19] These results are consistent with other studies that found mast-cell involvement in EIB.[20] The authors found that the mast-cell genes tryptase and carboxypeptidase A3 (CPA3) were significantly increased in EIB-positive asthmatics, but the expression of chymase was unaltered[19]; these findings are particularly note-worthy, because the appearance of secretory granule proteases is regulated by the peripheral tissue, and most prior studies have found that the mucosal mast cells ex-press tryptase, but not CPA3 or chymase.[21] This intraepithelial mast-cell phenotype with high expression of tryptase and CPA3, but low expression of chymase, was recently described in the T-helper type 2 (Th2) high phenotype of asthma.[22,23] Because this Th2 high phenotype is driven by interleukin (IL)-13,[24] it is interesting that a genetic study found an association between IL-13 gene polymorphisms and the severity of EIB, and with the treatment response to a $CysLT_1$ receptor antagonist among these subjects with EIB.[25] In making comparisons between asthmatics with and without EIB, the authors also identified a selective increase in the levels of the complement component C3a in individuals with EIB.[26] Thus, patients who are suscep-tible to EIB have epithelial shedding, overproduction of inflammatory mediators such as CysLTs, relative underproduction of protective lipid mediators, and infiltration of the airways with eosinophils and mast cells (**Fig. 1**).

INFLAMMATORY MEDIATOR RELEASE DURING EIB

During periods of high ventilation, large volumes of air are equilibrated to the humid-ified body conditions of the lower airways over a short period of time, leading to the transfer of water, with resulting stress to the epithelium and cooling of the airways, largely as a result of water transfer.[27–31] During tidal breathing at rest, little if any of the conditioning of the inspired air takes place beyond the upper airway and proximal trachea; however, conditioning of the inspired air takes place farther along the tracheobronchial tree as ventilation increases, forcing incompletely conditioned air to move deeply into the distal airways before it is brought to body conditions.[32] This movement of water out of the airways triggers the release of mediators predominantly from airway leukocytes. The cellular mechanism leading to the activation of leuko-cytes, either directly through the movement of water or via a signal from the epithelium in response to this water movement, is not known in detail. There is strong evidence that leukocyte-derived eicosanoids including CysLTs and PGD_2 are released into the airways following an exercise challenge as assessed by induced sputum analysis.[20,33] Similarly, in an analysis of EBC, the levels of CysLTs increased after exercise chal-lenge, most notably in the EIB-positive group; furthermore, the change in CysLTs in EBC following challenge was correlated with the severity of EIB.[34] In nonasthmatic

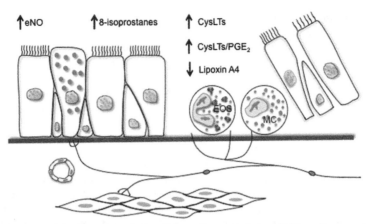

Fig. 1. Disease model of exercise-induced bronchoconstriction (EIB) pathogenesis. Studies examining differences between asthmatics with EIB to those without EIB have identified an increased concentration of shed epithelial cells, and infiltration of the airways with eosinophils and mast cells. There is an alteration in the balance of lipid mediators notable for an increase in cysteinyl leukotrienes (CysLTs), CysLT/prostaglandin E_2 (PGE$_2$) ratio, and 8-isoprostanes, and a reduction in lipoxin A4. eNO, exhaled nitric oxide. (*Adapted from* Hallstrand TS, Henderson WR Jr. Role of leukotrienes in exercise-induced bronchoconstriction. Curr Allergy Asthma Rep 2009;9:18–25.)

subjects, a gene-expression profiling study of peripheral blood following exercise challenge found increases in the expression of 5-lipoxygenase (5-LO) and 5-LO–activating protein (FLAP) in response to exercise challenge, as well as increased levels of LTs in the peripheral blood.[35]

The formation of LTs and other eicosanoids is initiated by the release of unesterified arachidonic acid by the hydrolysis at the sn-2 position of membrane phospholipids by phospholipase A_2 (PLA$_2$) (**Fig. 2**). Arachidonic acid is transferred by FLAP to 5-LO, initiating the oxygenation of arachidonic acid to 5(S)-hydroperoxyeicosatetraenoic acid (5S-HpETE), followed by dehydration to the unstable epoxide leukotriene A_4 (LTA$_4$).[36] The critical enzyme in the formation of CysLTs from LTA$_4$ is the enzyme LTC$_4$ synthase (LTC$_4$S), part of a family of membrane-bound proteins involved in eicosanoid and glutathione metabolism including FLAP, microsomal glutathione S-transferases (MGSTs), and microsomal prostaglandin E synthase 1. LTC$_4$S conjugates glutathione with a high degree of substrate selectivity for LTA$_4$,[37,38] leading to the generation of LTC$_4$ that is exported from the cell and rapidly metabolized to LTD$_4$ and then LTE$_4$.[39] The effects of LTD$_4$, including bronchoconstriction and airway inflammation, are mediated through the CysLT$_1$ receptor; however, the vast majority of CysLTs exist in the stable form of LTE$_4$ that does not interact with the CysLT$_1$ receptor.[39] Recent landmark studies have identified 2 different receptors for LTE$_4$ that participate in the development of allergic inflammation in animal models.[40] The incomplete effectiveness of CysLT1 receptor antagonists may be explained in part by the presence of these additional receptors for LTE$_4$.

Because the expression of 5-LO is largely restricted to myeloid cells, the majority of LT synthesis occurs in leukocytes; however, arachidonic acid and intermediates such as LTA$_4$ are permeable across cell membranes, allowing for the transcellular metabolism of eicosanoids. Several studies have demonstrated that eicosanoid production in leukocytes is increased when the leukocyte is cocultured with a structural cell such as an epithelial cell.[41] An important recent study demonstrated that 5-LO–deficient

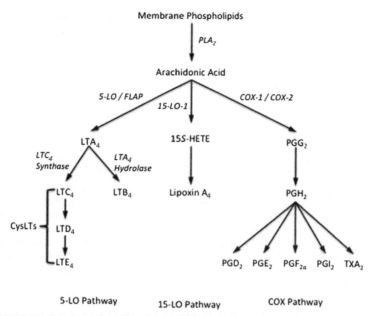

Fig. 2. Eicosanoid formation from arachidonic acid via the 5- and 15-lipoxygenase and cyclooxygenase pathways. COX, cyclooxygenase; CysLT, cysteinyl leukotriene; FLAP, 5-lipoxygenase–activating protein; HETE, hydroxyeicosatetraenoic acid; LO, lipoxygenase; PG, prostaglandin; PLA2, phospholipase A_2; TX, thromboxane.

mice transplanted with immune cells deficient in LTC_4S were able to make normal quantities of CysLTs, demonstrating that 5-LO–containing immune cells transfer intermediates that restore LT synthetic capacity by transcellular metabolism.[42]

The participation of epithelial cells in the release of mediators is suggested by several observations. First, the level of the epithelial-derived 15-lipoxygenase product 15S-hydroxyeicosatetranoic acid (15S-HETE) is increased after exercise challenge, and is elevated in asthmatics compared with controls after exercise challenge.[43] The other mechanism involves the relative underproduction of epithelial-derived PGE_2 in patients with EIB. Following exercise challenge the level of PGE_2 declines in the airways of asthmatics with EIB,[20] whereas PGE_2 tends to increase in normal subjects.[43] This relative imbalance in epithelial-derived PGE_2 when compared with leukocyte-derived LTs supports the hypothesis that transcellular transport of epithelial-derived arachidonic acid or a regulator of arachidonic acid release contributes to LT synthesis in leukocytes, favoring bronchoconstriction in the period following exercise challenge (**Fig. 3**).[43] One explanation for these findings is that the epithelium serves to activate the production of inflammatory eicosanoids by leukocytes that are in close contact, and that there is shunting of epithelial-derived arachidonic acid away from the epithelial-derived PGE_2. In cell culture, inflammatory cells cocultured with epithelial cells have increased synthesis of leukocyte-derived eicosanoids.[44] Under the influence of IL-13, epithelial cells have reduced capacity for PGE_2 synthesis through a reduction in the synthetic enzymes cyclooxygenase-2 (COX-2) and PGE synthase 1.[45] The underproduction of PGE_2 could also directly alter the formation of CysLTs and PGD_2, as inhaled PGE_2 regulates the levels of these eicosanoids after segmental allergen challenge[46] and PGE_2 directly alters CysLT formation in cultured mast cells.[47]

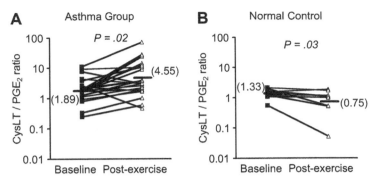

Fig. 3. Ratio of CysLTs to PGE$_2$ in induced sputum following exercise challenge. The levels of CysLTs and PGE$_2$ were measured in induced sputum in a group of asthmatics with EIB (*A*) and in a nonasthmatic control group (*B*) at baseline and after exercise challenge. The results demonstrate opposing effects of an increase in the CysLT/PGE$_2$ ratio after challenge in the asthma group, whereas the ratio decreased after challenge in the control group. (*Data from* Hallstrand TS, Chi EY, Singer AG, et al. Secreted phospholipase A2 group X overexpression in asthma and bronchial hyperresponsiveness. Am J Respir Crit Care Med 2007;176:1072–8.)

There is strong evidence that CysLTs play a causative role in the development of bronchoconstriction following exercise, through early proof-of-concept pharmacologic studies with CysLT$_1$ antagonists and 5-LO inhibitors. The CysLT$_1$ antagonist zafirlukast, given by inhalation to 9 patients with EIB 30 minutes before an exercise challenge, reduced the mean maximal percent decrease in FEV$_1$ to 14.5%, compared with 30.2% during placebo administration.[48] Oral zafirlukast was also shown to effectively inhibit EIB 2 hours after a single dose in a crossover study of 8 patients, resulting in a reduction in the mean maximal percent decrease in FEV$_1$ after challenge from 36.0% on placebo to 21.6% on zafirlukast.[49] A larger recent study showed that montelukast significantly reduced the severity of EIB at 2, 12, and 24 hours after a single dose, based on the maximum decrease in FEV$_1$ (10.8% montelukast vs 22.3% placebo at 2 hours, $P \leq .001$) and area under the curve for the percentage decrease in FEV$_1$.[50] A second similarly designed study of 62 patients with EIB also showed similar efficacy at 2 hours after a single dose of montelukast compared with placebo (11.7% montelukast vs 17.5% placebo, $P \leq .001$).[51] In a similar manner, the 5-LO inhibitor zileuton administered 4 times daily for 2 days reduced the decrease in FEV$_1$ after challenge, from 28.1% on placebo to 15.6% on zileuton.[52] These results clearly demonstrate a role for CysLTs in the pathogenesis of EIB but also indicate that the protection from EIB is incomplete, suggesting that mediators other than the CysLTs may play a significant role and that the loss of bronchoprotective mediators may be important. A recent study found that an ICS added to a CysLT$_1$ antagonist had improved efficacy over treatment with either an ICS or CysLT$_1$ antagonist alone.[53]

CELLULAR ACTIVATION DURING EIB

Mast cells and eosinophils are strongly implicated as the cellular sources of CysLTs and other eicosanoids such as PGD$_2$ in EIB. The eosinophil product eosinophilic cationic protein (ECP) is released into the airways following challenge, and the amount of ECP release varies with the severity of the EIB under different experimental conditions.[33] Following exercise challenge, histamine and the mast-cell protease tryptase are released into the airways, demonstrating mast-cell degranulation (**Fig. 4**).[20] Using

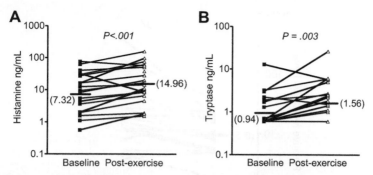

Fig. 4. Mast-cell degranulation following exercise challenge in asthmatics with EIB. The levels of histamine (*A*) and tryptase (*B*) were measured in induced sputum supernatant at baseline and on a separate day 30 minutes after exercise challenge. Significant increases in both histamine and tryptase were observed following exercise challenge in subjects with EIB. (*Data from* Hallstrand TS, Moody MW, Wurfel MM, et al. Inflammatory basis of exercise-induced bronchoconstriction. Am J Respir Crit Care Med 2005;172:679–86.)

the urinary levels of $9\alpha,11\beta$-PGF_2 as a marker of PGD_2 metabolism and mast-cell activation in response to EVH, the release of PGD_2 can be inhibited by pretreatment with a cromone or a high dose of inhaled steroid, suggesting that PGD_2 release by mast cells may play an important role in the development of bronchoconstriction after exercise challenge.[13,54] Using mannitol challenge as a surrogate for exercise, pharmacologic inhibitors indicate that histamine is responsible for bronchoconstriction early after challenge while the release of CysLTs is responsible for sustained bronchoconstriction.[55]

CONTRIBUTION OF SENSORY NERVES

Sensory nerves release neurokinins when activated through a process called retrograde axonal transmission, leading to bronchoconstriction and mucus release. There is evidence in animal models that the production of eicosanoids such as CysLTs mediate bronchoconstriction, at least in part through the activation of airway sensory nerves. Although sensory nerves may be activated directly by osmotic stimuli, several eicosanoids can either directly activate or alter the activation threshold of sensory nerves.[56] In a dog model, a combination neurokinin-1 and neurokinin-2 receptor antagonist inhibited hyperpnea-induced bronchoconstriction (HIB) and the generation of LTs that are known in this model to cause HIB.[57] In a guinea pig model of HIB, either a 5-LO inhibitor or a CysLT$_1$ antagonist inhibited HIB and the release of neurokinins, whereas a neurokinin-2 receptor antagonist inhibited HIB but not the release of leukotrienes, suggesting that leukotrienes cause bronchoconstriction via sensory nerves during HIB.[58] In humans, the effects of neurokinin-1 antagonists have been modest[59,60]; however, this lack of efficacy may be due to the predominance of neurokinin A, which binds predominantly to the neurokinin-2 receptor.[61] As goblet-cell mucin release is initiated via neurokinin release, it is notable that mucin 5AC (MUC5AC), the predominant gel-forming mucin of goblet cells, is released into the airways during EIB in humans (**Fig. 5**) and is associated with the levels of CysLTs in the airways.[62] Furthermore, the levels of neurokinin A and CysLTs in these individuals after exercise challenge are correlated, suggesting that CysLTs mediate the activation of sensory nerves and mucus release during EIB in humans.[62]

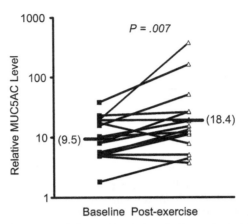

Fig. 5. Goblet cell mucin release following exercise challenge in asthmatics with EIB. The levels of the gel-forming mucin MUC5AC were measured before and after exercise challenge in induced sputum supernatant in subjects with EIB. The induced sputum samples were dialyzed to remove the dithiothreitol (DTT) before analysis. A significant increase in MUC5AC was observed following exercise challenge. (*Data from* Hallstrand TS, Debley JS, Farin FM, et al. Role of MUC5AC in the pathogenesis of exercise-induced bronchoconstriction. J Allergy Clin Immunol 2007;119:1092–8.)

LATE PHASE RESPONSE

Despite the very compelling evidence that exercise challenge acutely causes the release of inflammatory mediators into the airways, several studies failed to demonstrate a cellular influx into the airways or an increase in direct AHR following an exercise challenge.[63–66] A physiologic late-phase response has also been difficult to demonstrate in many studies, or has been attributed to factors such as the inevitable fluctuation in airway tone among patients with asthma.[67–69] Despite this controversy, some studies indicate that a portion of patients have a second wave of airflow obstruction consistent with a late-phase response to exercise challenge,[70,71] and there is clearly a late-phase response in a dog model of HIB.[72] The late-phase response to exercise challenge may also be inhibited by treatment with the CysLT$_1$ receptor antagonist montelukast.[70] Recent provocative results using EBC demonstrate an increase in high-sensitivity C-reactive protein only in asthmatics with EIB following exercise challenge.[73] In addition, the F$_{ENO}$, serum ECP, and AHR to inhaled histamine were all increased following exercise challenge in asthmatics with EIB.[73] Further, RANTES and eotaxin in EBC were increased in asthmatics relative to controls, and the levels of RANTES and eotaxin were increased in EBC after exercise challenge in the group with EIB but not in asthmatics without EIB.[74,75] These data indicate that inflammatory mediator release with exercise challenge may recruit leukocytes to the airways, but the magnitude of such leukocyte recruitment is small or counterregulated by anti-inflammatory pathways.

REGULATION OF EICOSANOID PRODUCTION AND LEUKOCYTE ACTIVATION BY THE EPITHELIUM

A unifying concept regarding the pathogenesis of EIB is that the epithelium may regulate the response to water loss experienced during exercise challenge. One possibility is that a regulator of eicosanoid formation is released by the airway epithelium in response to water loss. Water is transferred out of the airways during exercise, leading to the movement of water by the semipermeable and osmotically sensitive epithelium that rapidly corrects alterations in airway surface liquid (ASL) osmolarity (**Fig. 6**).[76] A similar epithelial response with the transfer of water should occur in response to exogenous osmolar stimuli such as mannitol and hypertonic saline. In response to water loss in the luminal surface, epithelial cell height reduces as the cells transfer water to the surface.[77,78] Because of the ability of the epithelium to respond to movement of water, there is little evidence that any osmotic gradient exists more than transiently in the ASL.[79] However, evaporative water loss from epithelial cells initiates the release of cellular adenosine triphosphate and adenosine, leading to the activation of chloride channels and increasing intracellular calcium.[76] This stress to the epithelium during exercise may explain the increased levels of adenosine in EBC following exercise challenge that correlate with the severity of EIB.[80] It is also known that osmotic stimuli can directly activate inflammatory cells such as mast cells[81]; however, hyperosmolarity per se exists only transiently in the airways, and likely serves as a stimulus primarily to the epithelium. The connection between epithelial stress induced by water loss and the activation of leukocytes in the airways needs to be understood more completely.

The first rate-limiting step in eicosanoid formation is the release of arachidonic acid mediated by PLA_2. It is well known that cytosolic $PLA_2\alpha$ ($cPLA_2\alpha$) functions as a major regulator of efficient eicosanoid synthesis.[82] More recently, a family of secreted PLA_2s ($sPLA_2$) have been described that can also serve as regulators of eicosanoid synthesis and may preferentially direct eicosanoid production toward LT synthesis.[39] It has been known for some time that $sPLA_2$ activity in the airways increases following allergen challenge in the upper and lower airways.[83–85] Of the mammalian $sPLA_2$s, groups V and X have generated the most interest because of their capacity to initiate cellular eicosanoid synthesis,[86] particularly $sPLA_2$ group X ($sPLA_2$-X), because it is the most potent of the $sPLA_2$s at releasing arachidonic acid from membrane phospholipids. In murine models of asthma, genetic deficiency of either $sPLA_2$-V or $sPLA_2$-X attenuates the development of allergen-induced inflammation, mucus release, and AHR,[87,88] as does the pharmacologic inhibition of human $sPLA_2$-X expressed in a transgenic

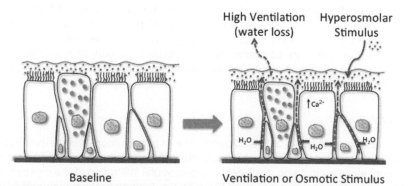

Fig. 6. Basic overview of the epithelial response to water loss from the airway surface liquid. As ventilation increases, water is lost from the airway surface liquid, resulting in transient hyperosmolarity and the passive movement of water from airway epithelial cells (*arrows*) to restore the osmolarity of the airway surface liquid. The movement of water causes epithelial cells to shrink and initiates cellular signaling events, including an increase in intracellular calcium (Ca^{2+}). The addition of osmotically active substances such as mannitol and hypertonic saline similarly cause water movement to restore the surface osmolarity.

mouse model.[89] The authors have found that $sPLA_2$-X levels are increased in the bronchoalveolar lavage fluid of patients with asthma and that $sPLA_2$-X is predominantly expressed in the airway epithelium.[90] In addition, using semiquantitative techniques they have found that $sPLA_2$-X protein in induced sputum supernatant and epithelial cells immunostaining for $sPLA_2$-X in induced sputum increases following exercise challenge, suggesting that activation or release of $sPLA_2$-X may be involved in the generation of eicosanoids following exercise challenge.[43]

The release of $sPLA_2$-X or other similar enzymes into the airways after exercise challenge could play an important role in the pathogenesis of EIB through the initiation of mediator formation in leukocytes, the degradation of surfactant phospholipids, and the generation of lysophospholipids. The authors examined the ability of $sPLA_2$-X to efficiently activate CysLT formation by human eosinophils.[91] Recombinant human $sPLA_2$-X initiates arachidonic acid release and CysLT synthesis through a mechanism that is dependent on the enzymatic activity of $sPLA_2$-X, but could also be replicated by lysophospholipids released by eosinophils in response to $sPLA_2$-X. Of interest, the full mechanism of $sPLA_2$-X–mediated activation of eosinophils involves the activation of the mitogen-activated kinase cascade and the activation of $cPLA_2\alpha$; however, CysLT formation is amplified by $sPLA_2$-X, probably as an additional source of arachidonic acid.

Another important finding is the increased expression of transglutaminase 2 (TGM2) in the airways of patients with EIB relative to asthmatics without EIB.[19] It is notable that the TGM2 gene is located on chromosome 20q11.2-12 near a cluster of genes related to epithelial barrier function, in close proximity to a region linked to both atopic dermatitis and asthma.[92] Using an in vitro assay of $sPLA_2$ activity, the authors found that recombinant human TGM2 enzymatically modifies $sPLA_2$-X, leading to a substantial increase in the $sPLA_2$ activity of the enzyme, suggesting that one of the mechanisms of TGM2 action in asthma is regulation of eicosanoid and lysophospholipid synthesis. The potential importance of this finding was highlighted in mouse models showing that TGM2 is induced in the airways of mice sensitized and challenged with ovalbumin in the presence of adjuvant,[93] as well as in mouse models of PMA-induced atopic dermatitis and immunoglobulin E (IgE)-dependent passive cutaneous anaphylaxis.[94] In one study a peptide that inhibits both TGM2 and PLA_2 reduced allergen-induced airway inflammation and eicosanoid formation, but the specific role of TGM2 remains to be fully elucidated.[93] A chemical inhibitor of TGM2 partially inhibited PMA-induced dermatitis and IgE-dependent cutaneous anaphylaxis.[94] Collectively these studies suggest that the epithelium can serve as an important regulator of eicosanoid formation, and that the release of $sPLA_2$-X from the airway epithelium could regulate mediator formation in EIB.

SUMMARY

Exercise challenge leads to a distinct syndrome of bronchoconstriction that occurs in a susceptible group of subjects who have epithelial shedding, overproduction of inflammatory eicosanoids, and mast-cell and eosinophil infiltration of the airways. Exercise challenge causes water loss from the airways, leading to the movement of water from the epithelium to correct the resultant transient shift in osmolarity. Although the precise mechanism by which water loss leads to the activation of leukocytes is not known, it is clear that exercise challenge initiates the release of inflammatory mediators from leukocytes such as mast cells and eosinophils. In the case of the release of CysLTs, it is clear that the release of CysLTs acts via the $CysLT_1$ receptor to initiate bronchoconstriction, based on studies in humans using pharmacologic inhibitors.

Other mediators such as 15S-HETE and PGD_2 are released from the airway cells, but the specific role of these mediators in the development of bronchoconstriction is less certain. Based predominantly on animal and in vitro studies, sensory nerves seem to play an important role in either transmitting the effects of eicosanoids that are released in the airways or as direct sensors of changes in airway osmolarity, a process that is potentiated by elevated levels of eicosanoids. A possible explanation for the cellular events in the airways is that the airway epithelium, acting as the primary sensor of water loss, releases a product that serves to activate leukocytes that are in close contact with the epithelium, leading to the release of leukocyte-derived eicosanoids and activation of sensory nerves. One such product is $sPLA_2$-X, which is avidly expressed in the airway epithelium, increased in the airway fluid of asthmatics, and serves to activate airway cells such as eosinophils to generate CysLTs. The regulation of these cellular events requires further study so that targeted therapies may be developed to modulate this important aspect of asthma.

REFERENCES

1. Joos GF, O'Connor B, Anderson SD, et al. Indirect airway challenges. Eur Respir J 2003;21:1050–68.
2. Carraro S, Corradi M, Zanconato S, et al. Exhaled breath condensate cysteinyl leukotrienes are increased in children with exercise-induced bronchoconstriction. J Allergy Clin Immunol 2005;115:764–70.
3. Cabral AL, Conceicao GM, Fonseca-Guedes CH, et al. Exercise-induced bronchospasm in children: effects of asthma severity. Am J Respir Crit Care Med 1999;159:1819–23.
4. Hallstrand TS, Moody MW, Aitken ML, et al. Airway immunopathology of asthma with exercise-induced bronchoconstriction. J Allergy Clin Immunol 2005;116: 586–93.
5. Freezer NJ, Croasdell H, Doull IJ, et al. Effect of regular inhaled beclomethasone on exercise and methacholine airway responses in school children with recurrent wheeze. Eur Respir J 1995;8:1488–93.
6. Holzer K, Anderson SD, Douglass J. Exercise in elite summer athletes: challenges for diagnosis. J Allergy Clin Immunol 2002;110:374–80.
7. Frank PI, Morris JA, Hazell ML, et al. Long term prognosis in preschool children with wheeze: longitudinal postal questionnaire study 1993-2004. BMJ 2008;336: 1423–6.
8. Riiser A, Hovland V, Carlsen KH, et al. Does bronchial hyperresponsiveness in childhood predict active asthma in adolescence? Am J Respir Crit Care Med 2012;186:493–500.
9. Stern DA, Morgan WJ, Halonen M, et al. Wheezing and bronchial hyperresponsiveness in early childhood as predictors of newly diagnosed asthma in early adulthood: a longitudinal birth-cohort study. Lancet 2008;372:1058–64.
10. Joshi S, Powell T, Watkins WJ, et al. Exercise-induced bronchoconstriction in school-aged children who had chronic lung disease in infancy. J Pediatr 2012. [Epub ahead of print].
11. Scollo M, Zanconato S, Ongaro R, et al. Exhaled nitric oxide and exercise-induced bronchoconstriction in asthmatic children. Am J Respir Crit Care Med 2000;161:1047–50.
12. Malmberg LP, Pelkonen AS, Mattila PS, et al. Exhaled nitric oxide and exercise-induced bronchoconstriction in young wheezy children—interactions with atopy. Pediatr Allergy Immunol 2009;20:673–8.

13. Kippelen P, Larsson J, Anderson SD, et al. Effect of sodium cromoglycate on mast cell mediators during hyperpnea in athletes. Med Sci Sports Exerc 2010; 42:1853–60.

14. Barreto M, Villa MP, Olita C, et al. 8-Isoprostane in exhaled breath condensate and exercise-induced bronchoconstriction in asthmatic children and adolescents. Chest 2009;135:66–73.

15. Tahan F, Saraymen R, Gumus H. The role of lipoxin A4 in exercise-induced bronchoconstriction in asthma. J Asthma 2008;45:161–4.

16. Melillo E, Woolley KL, Manning PJ, et al. Effect of inhaled PGE_2 on exercise-induced bronchoconstriction in asthmatic subjects. Am J Respir Crit Care Med 1994;149:1138–41.

17. Cai Y, Bjermer L, Halstensen TS. Bronchial mast cells are the dominating LTC4S-expressing cells in aspirin-tolerant asthma. Am J Respir Cell Mol Biol 2003;29: 683–93.

18. Duong M, Subbarao P, Adelroth E, et al. Sputum eosinophils and the response of exercise-induced bronchoconstriction to corticosteroid in asthma. Chest 2008; 133:404–11.

19. Hallstrand TS, Wurfel MM, Lai Y, et al. Transglutaminase 2, a novel regulator of eicosanoid production in asthma revealed by genome-wide expression profiling of distinct asthma phenotypes. PLoS One 2010;5:e8583.

20. Hallstrand TS, Moody MW, Wurfel MM, et al. Inflammatory basis of exercise-induced bronchoconstriction. Am J Respir Crit Care Med 2005;172:679–86.

21. Gurish MF, Austen KF. Developmental origin and functional specialization of mast cell subsets. Immunity 2012;37:25–33.

22. Dougherty RH, Sidhu SS, Raman K, et al. Accumulation of intraepithelial mast cells with a unique protease phenotype in T(h)2-high asthma. J Allergy Clin Immunol 2010;125:1046–1053.e8.

23. Woodruff PG, Boushey HA, Dolganov GM, et al. Genome-wide profiling identifies epithelial cell genes associated with asthma and with treatment response to corticosteroids. Proc Natl Acad Sci U S A 2007;104:15858–63.

24. Woodruff PG, Modrek B, Choy DF, et al. T-helper type 2-driven inflammation defines major subphenotypes of asthma. Am J Respir Crit Care Med 2009;180: 388–95.

25. Kang MJ, Lee SY, Kim HB, et al. Association of IL-13 polymorphisms with leukotriene receptor antagonist drug responsiveness in Korean children with exercise-induced bronchoconstriction. Pharmacogenet Genomics 2008;18:551–8.

26. Gharib SA, Nguyen EV, Lai Y, et al. Induced sputum proteome in healthy subjects and asthmatic patients. J Allergy Clin Immunol 2011;128:1176–1184.e6.

27. Anderson SD, Schoeffel RE. Respiratory heat and water loss during exercise in patients with asthma. Effect of repeated exercise challenge. Eur J Respir Dis 1982;63:472–80.

28. Anderson SD, Schoeffel RE, Black JL, et al. Airway cooling as the stimulus to exercise-induced asthma—a re-evaluation. Eur J Respir Dis 1985;67:20–30.

29. Gilbert IA, McFadden ER Jr. Airway cooling and rewarming. The second reaction sequence in exercise-induced asthma. J Clin Invest 1992;90:699–704.

30. Strauss RH, McFadden ER Jr, Ingram RH Jr, et al. Influence of heat and humidity on the airway obstruction induced by exercise in asthma. J Clin Invest 1978;61: 433–40.

31. Deal EC Jr, McFadden ER Jr, Ingram RH Jr, et al. Role of respiratory heat exchange in production of exercise-induced asthma. J Appl Physiol 1979;46: 467–75.

32. Gilbert IA, Fouke JM, McFadden ER Jr. Heat and water flux in the intrathoracic airways and exercise-induced asthma. J Appl Physiol 1987;63:1681–91.
33. Mickleborough TD, Lindley MR, Ray S. Dietary salt, airway inflammation, and diffusion capacity in exercise-induced asthma. Med Sci Sports Exerc 2005;37: 904–14.
34. Bikov A, Gajdocsi R, Huszar E, et al. Exercise increases exhaled breath condensate cysteinyl leukotriene concentration in asthmatic patients. J Asthma 2010;47: 1057–62.
35. Hilberg T, Deigner HP, Moller E, et al. Transcription in response to physical stress—clues to the molecular mechanisms of exercise-induced asthma. FASEB J 2005;19:1492–4.
36. Mandal AK, Jones PB, Bair AM, et al. The nuclear membrane organization of leukotriene synthesis. Proc Natl Acad Sci U S A 2008;105:20434–9.
37. Ago H, Kanaoka Y, Irikura D, et al. Crystal structure of a human membrane protein involved in cysteinyl leukotriene biosynthesis. Nature 2007;448:609–12.
38. Martinez Molina D, Wetterholm A, Kohl A, et al. Structural basis for synthesis of inflammatory mediators by human leukotriene c_4 synthase. Nature 2007;448: 613–6.
39. Hallstrand TS, Henderson WR Jr. An update on the role of leukotrienes in asthma. Curr Opin Allergy Clin Immunol 2010;10:60–6.
40. Austen KF, Maekawa A, Kanaoka Y, et al. The leukotriene E4 puzzle: finding the missing pieces and revealing the pathobiologic implications. J Allergy Clin Immunol 2009;124:406–14 [quiz: 415–6].
41. Holgate ST, Peters-Golden M, Panettieri RA, et al. Roles of cysteinyl leukotrienes in airway inflammation, smooth muscle function, and remodeling. J Allergy Clin Immunol 2003;111:S18–34.
42. Zarini S, Gijon MA, Ransome AE, et al. Transcellular biosynthesis of cysteinyl leukotrienes in vivo during mouse peritoneal inflammation. Proc Natl Acad Sci U S A 2009;106:8296–301.
43. Hallstrand TS, Chi EY, Singer AG, et al. Secreted phospholipase A2 group X overexpression in asthma and bronchial hyperresponsiveness. Am J Respir Crit Care Med 2007;176:1072–8.
44. Wijewickrama GT, Kim JH, Kim YJ, et al. Systematic evaluation of transcellular activities of secretory phospholipases A_2. High activity of group V phospholipases A_2 to induce eicosanoid biosynthesis in neighboring inflammatory cells. J Biol Chem 2006;281:10935–44.
45. Trudeau J, Hu H, Chibana K, et al. Selective downregulation of prostaglandin E_2-related pathways by the Th2 cytokine IL-13. J Allergy Clin Immunol 2006; 117:1446–54.
46. Hartert TV, Dworski RT, Mellen BG, et al. Prostaglandin E_2 decreases allergen-stimulated release of prostaglandin D_2 in airways of subjects with asthma. Am J Respir Crit Care Med 2000;162:637–40.
47. Feng C, Beller EM, Bagga S, et al. Human mast cells express multiple EP receptors for prostaglandin E that differentially modulate activation responses. Blood 2006;107:3243–50.
48. Makker HK, Lau LC, Thomson HW, et al. The protective effect of inhaled leukotriene D_4 receptor antagonist ICI 204,219 against exercise-induced asthma. Am Rev Respir Dis 1993;147:1413–8.
49. Finnerty JP, Wood-Baker R, Thomson H, et al. Role of leukotrienes in exercise-induced asthma. Inhibitory effect of ICI 204219, a potent leukotriene D_4 receptor antagonist. Am Rev Respir Dis 1992;145:746–9.

50. Pearlman DS, van Adelsberg J, Philip G, et al. Onset and duration of protection against exercise-induced bronchoconstriction by a single oral dose of montelukast. Ann Allergy Asthma Immunol 2006;97:98–104.
51. Philip G, Villaran C, Pearlman DS, et al. Protection against exercise-induced bronchoconstriction two hours after a single oral dose of montelukast. J Asthma 2007; 44:213–7.
52. Meltzer SS, Hasday JD, Cohn J, et al. Inhibition of exercise-induced bronchospasm by zileuton: a 5-lipoxygenase inhibitor. Am J Respir Crit Care Med 1996;153:931–5.
53. Duong M, Amin R, Baatjes AJ, et al. The effect of montelukast, budesonide alone, and in combination on exercise-induced bronchoconstriction. J Allergy Clin Immunol 2012;130:535–539.e3.
54. Kippelen P, Larsson J, Anderson SD, et al. Acute effects of beclomethasone on hyperpnea-induced bronchoconstriction. Med Sci Sports Exerc 2010;42:273–80.
55. Currie GP, Haggart K, Lee DK, et al. Effects of mediator antagonism on mannitol and adenosine monophosphate challenges. Clin Exp Allergy 2003;33:783–8.
56. Taylor-Clark TE, Nassenstein C, Undem BJ. Leukotriene D increases the excitability of capsaicin-sensitive nasal sensory nerves to electrical and chemical stimuli. Br J Pharmacol 2008;154:1359–68.
57. Freed AN, McCulloch S, Meyers T, et al. Neurokinins modulate hyperventilation-induced bronchoconstriction in canine peripheral airways. Am J Respir Crit Care Med 2003;167:1102–8.
58. Lai YL, Lee SP. Mediators in hyperpnea-induced bronchoconstriction of guinea pigs. Naunyn Schmiedebergs Arch Pharmacol 1999;360:597–602.
59. Fahy JV, Wong HH, Geppetti P, et al. Effect of an NK1 receptor antagonist (CP-99,994) on hypertonic saline-induced bronchoconstriction and cough in male asthmatic subjects. Am J Respir Crit Care Med 1995;152:879–84.
60. Ichinose M, Miura M, Yamauchi H, et al. A neurokinin 1-receptor antagonist improves exercise-induced airway narrowing in asthmatic patients. Am J Respir Crit Care Med 1996;153:936–41.
61. Barnes PJ. Neurogenic inflammation in the airways. Respir Physiol 2001;125: 145–54.
62. Hallstrand TS, Debley JS, Farin FM, et al. Role of MUC5AC in the pathogenesis of exercise-induced bronchoconstriction. J Allergy Clin Immunol 2007;119:1092–8.
63. Foresi A, Mattoli S, Corbo GM, et al. Late bronchial response and increase in methacholine hyperresponsiveness after exercise and distilled water challenge in atopic subjects with asthma with dual asthmatic response to allergen inhalation. J Allergy Clin Immunol 1986;78:1130–9.
64. Gauvreau GM, Ronnen GM, Watson RM, et al. Exercise-induced bronchoconstriction does not cause eosinophilic airway inflammation or airway hyperresponsiveness in subjects with asthma. Am J Respir Crit Care Med 2000;162: 1302–7.
65. Jarjour NN, Calhoun WJ. Exercise-induced asthma is not associated with mast cell activation or airway inflammation. J Allergy Clin Immunol 1992;89:60–8.
66. Zawadski DK, Lenner KA, McFadden ER Jr. Effect of exercise on nonspecific airway reactivity in asthmatics. J Appl Physiol 1988;64:812–6.
67. Boner AL, Vallone G, Chiesa M, et al. Reproducibility of late phase pulmonary response to exercise and its relationship to bronchial hyperreactivity in children with chronic asthma. Pediatr Pulmonol 1992;14:156–9.
68. Iikura Y, Inui H, Obata T, et al. Drug effects on exercise-induced late asthmatic responses. N Engl Reg Allergy Proc 1988;9:203–7.

69. Zawadski DK, Lenner KA, McFadden ER Jr. Re-examination of the late asthmatic response to exercise. Am Rev Respir Dis 1988;137:837–41.
70. Melo RE, Sole D, Naspitz CK. Exercise-induced bronchoconstriction in children: montelukast attenuates the immediate-phase and late-phase responses. J Allergy Clin Immunol 2003;111:301–7.
71. Crimi E, Balbo A, Milanese M, et al. Airway inflammation and occurrence of delayed bronchoconstriction in exercise-induced asthma. Am Rev Respir Dis 1992;146:507–12.
72. Freed AN, Bromberger-Barnea B, Menkes HA. Dry air-induced constriction in lung periphery: a canine model of exercise-induced asthma. J Appl Physiol 1985;59:1986–90.
73. Zietkowski Z, Skiepko R, Tomasiak-Lozowska MM, et al. Changes in high-sensitivity C-reactive protein in serum and exhaled breath condensate after intensive exercise in patients with allergic asthma. Int Arch Allergy Immunol 2010;153:75–85.
74. Zietkowski Z, Skiepko R, Tomasiak-Lozowska MM, et al. RANTES in exhaled breath condensate of allergic asthma patients with exercise-induced bronchoconstriction. Respiration 2010;80:463–71.
75. Zietkowski Z, Skiepko R, Tomasiak-Lozowska MM, et al. Eotaxin in exhaled breath condensate of allergic asthma patients with exercise-induced bronchoconstriction. Respiration 2011;82:169–76.
76. Tarran R. Regulation of airway surface liquid volume and mucus transport by active ion transport. Proc Am Thorac Soc 2004;1:42–6.
77. Matsui H, Davis CW, Tarran R, et al. Osmotic water permeabilities of cultured, well-differentiated normal and cystic fibrosis airway epithelia. J Clin Invest 2000;105:1419–27.
78. Willumsen NJ, Davis CW, Boucher RC. Selective response of human airway epithelia to luminal but not serosal solution hypertonicity. Possible role for proximal airway epithelia as an osmolality transducer. J Clin Invest 1994;94:779–87.
79. Kotaru C, Hejal RB, Finigan JH, et al. Desiccation and hypertonicity of the airway surface fluid and thermally induced asthma. J Appl Physiol 2003;94:227–33.
80. Csoma Z, Huszar E, Vizi E, et al. Adenosine level in exhaled breath increases during exercise-induced bronchoconstriction. Eur Respir J 2005;25:873–8.
81. Gulliksson M, Palmberg L, Nilsson G, et al. Release of prostaglandin D_2 and leukotriene C_4 in response to hyperosmolar stimulation of mast cells. Allergy 2006;61:1473–9.
82. Uozumi N, Kume K, Nagase T, et al. Role of cytosolic phospholipase A_2 in allergic response and parturition. Nature 1997;390:618–22.
83. Bowton DL, Seeds MC, Fasano MB, et al. Phospholipase A_2 and arachidonate increase in bronchoalveolar lavage fluid after inhaled antigen challenge in asthmatics. Am J Respir Crit Care Med 1997;155:421–5.
84. Chilton FH, Averill FJ, Hubbard WC, et al. Antigen-induced generation of lysophospholipids in human airways. J Exp Med 1996;183:2235–45.
85. Stadel JM, Hoyle K, Naclerio RM, et al. Characterization of phospholipase A_2 from human nasal lavage. Am J Respir Cell Mol Biol 1994;11:108–13.
86. Singer AG, Ghomashchi F, Le Calvez C, et al. Interfacial kinetic and binding properties of the complete set of human and mouse groups I, II, V, X, and XII secreted phospholipases a_2. J Biol Chem 2002;277:48535–49.
87. Henderson WR Jr, Chi EY, Bollinger JG, et al. Importance of group X-secreted phospholipase A_2 in allergen-induced airway inflammation and remodeling in a mouse asthma model. J Exp Med 2007;204:865–77.

88. Munoz NM, Meliton AY, Arm JP, et al. Deletion of secretory group V phospholipase A attenuates cell migration and airway hyperresponsiveness in immunosensitized mice. J Immunol 2007;179:4800–7.

89. Hendersen WR Jr, Oslund RC, Bollinger JG, et al. Blockade of human group X secreted phospholipase A-induced airway inflammation and hyperresponsiveness in a mouse asthma model by a selective group X secreted phospholipase A inhibitor. J Biol Chem 2011;286:28049–55.

90. Hallstrand TS, Lai Y, Ni Z, et al. Relationship between levels of secreted phospholipase A groups IIA and X in the airways and asthma severity. Clin Exp Allergy 2011;41:801–10.

91. Lai Y, Oslund RC, Bollinger JG, et al. Eosinophil cysteinyl leukotriene synthesis mediated by exogenous secreted phospholipase A group X. J Biol Chem 2010;285:41491–500.

92. Cookson W. The immunogenetics of asthma and eczema: a new focus on the epithelium. Nat Rev Immunol 2004;4:978–88.

93. Kim DY, Park BS, Hong GU, et al. Anti-inflammatory effects of the R2 peptide, an inhibitor of transglutaminase 2, in a mouse model of allergic asthma, induced by ovalbumin. Br J Pharmacol 2011;162:210–25.

94. Kim Y, Eom S, Kim K, et al. Transglutaminase II interacts with RAC1, regulates production of reactive oxygen species, expression of snail, secretion of Th2 cytokines and mediates in vitro and in vivo allergic inflammation. Mol Immunol 2010;47:1010–22.

Refractoriness to Exercise Challenge

A Review of the Mechanisms Old and New

Johan Larsson, MD[a,b,c,*], Sandra D. Anderson, PhD, DSc, MD(Hon)[d],
Sven-Erik Dahlén, MD, PhD[b,c], Barbro Dahlén, MD, PhD[a,c]

KEYWORDS

- Asthma • Exercise • Refractoriness • Leukotriene • Prostaglandin

KEY POINTS

- Exercise-induced bronchoconstriction is defined as a decrease in forced expiratory volume in 1 second of 10% to 15% or more and is seen in most patients with asthma.
- Refractoriness, a decreased responsiveness to repeated exercise challenge, is an inborn protective mechanism with an unknown mechanism of development.
- Refractoriness is not associated with decreased levels of the primary mediators of bronchoconstriction, cysteinyl leukotrienes, or prostaglandin D_2, as previously suggested.
- Desensitization of the cysteinyl leukotriene receptor ($CysLT_1$) through interplay between leukotrienes and prostaglandins is suggested as a possible mechanism for refractoriness.

INTRODUCTION

"Exercise-induced bronchoconstriction (EIB) and exercise induced asthma are the terms used to describe the transient increase in airways resistance that follows vigorous exercise."[1] Most untreated patients with asthma will experience bronchoconstriction after exercise,[2–4] and the prevalence of positive responses in those being

Funding Sources: J. Larsson, B. Dahlén, S-E. Dahlén: Karolinska Institutet, the Center for Allergy Research and the Stockholm County Council (ALF), and the following Swedish foundations: Heart Lung Foundation, Association Against Asthma and Allergy, Medical Research Council, and Vinnova (CiDAT). S.D. Anderson: None.
Conflicts of Interest: Nil.
[a] Lung and Allergy Research, Division of Respiratory Medicine and Allergy, Department of Medicine, Karolinska University Hospital Huddinge, Karolinska Institutet, M53, 14186 Stockholm, Sweden; [b] Division of Physiology, The National Institute of Environmental Medicine, Karolinska Institutet, Box 287, 17177 Stockholm, Sweden; [c] Centre for Allergy Research, Karolinska Institutet, Karolinska Institutet, Box 287, 17177 Stockholm, Sweden; [d] Department of Respiratory and Sleep Medicine, Royal Prince Alfred Hospital, E11, Missenden Road, Camperdown, New South Wales 2050, Australia
* Corresponding author. Lung and Allergy Research, Department of Medicine, Karolinska University Hospital Huddinge, Karolinska Institutet, M53, 14186 Stockholm, Sweden.
E-mail address: Johan.Larsson@ki.se

Immunol Allergy Clin N Am 33 (2013) 329–345
http://dx.doi.org/10.1016/j.iac.2013.02.004
0889-8561/13/$ – see front matter © 2013 Elsevier Inc. All rights reserved.

treated with inhaled corticosteroids is about 50%.[5,6] EIB is identified by measuring a decrease in forced expiratory volume in the first second of expiration (FEV_1) after exercise of at least 10% to 15% from the pre-exercise value. Recovery of the FEV_1 normally occurs within 30 to 60 minutes but can be aided by inhaling a β_2-agonist. Most of those with EIB are atopic.[7,8] Late asthmatic responses are very uncommon, if ever present following EIB.[9,10]

When the same exercise challenge is repeated within 1 hour, about 50% of patients with asthma will demonstrate less than half the response they had on the initial challenge, as measured by a decrease in FEV_1 or peak expiratory flow (**Fig. 1**).[11,12] This decreased response to repeated challenges is called *refractoriness* and its duration is called the *refractory period*. To avoid false identification of refractoriness, it is essential that the lung function returns to close to the baseline value before the challenge is repeated (see **Fig. 1**). The precise mechanism for refractoriness is not known, although there have been several proposals from studies performed in patients with clinically

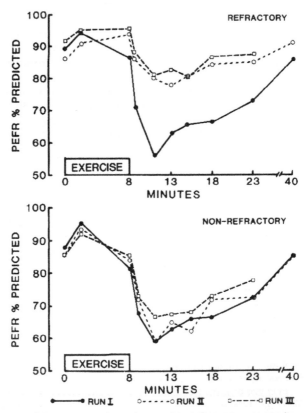

Fig. 1. Bronchoconstrictive response in patients with asthma on repeated exercise challenge. Peak expiratory flow rate (PEFR) expressed as a percentage of the predicted normal value before, during, and after 3 exercise challenges separated by 40 minutes in 16 patients with asthma. PEFR has now been replaced by FEV_1 as the lung function test to measure EIB. The patients included all returned to within 10% of baseline lung function before the start of the subsequent challenge. Refractoriness was seen in 8 patients, whereas no protection was seen in 8 patients. (*From* Schoeffel RE, Anderson SD, Gillam I, et al. Multiple exercise and histamine challenge in asthmatic patients. Thorax 1980;35:164–70; with permission.)

recognized asthma over the last 30 years. Identification of this protective mechanism is advantageous, first, because it has the potential to improve control and resolution of one of the most common causes of an attack of asthma and, second, because elucidation of the mechanism also has the potential to introduce a new target for treatment of asthma in general. The authors have reviewed the current clinical investigations into the stimulus and mechanism of EIB and the previously proposed mechanisms for refractoriness. The mechanism most generally accepted involves the release of a protective prostaglandin (PG), presumably PGE_2, during the first challenge. This mechanism has, however, not been conclusively established. Considering these earlier observations and some recent observations, the authors propose desensitization of the G protein–coupled cysteinyl leukotriene receptor$_1$ ($CysLT_1$) as the mechanism of refractoriness and that this desensitization is the effect of interplay between leukotrienes (LTs) and PGs.

WHY DOES EXERCISE PROVOKE AN ATTACK OF ASTHMA?

The most important determinants of EIB are the ventilation reached and sustained during exercise and the water content and temperature of the inspired air. The higher the ventilation reached and the drier the air inspired, the greater the potential to provoke bronchoconstriction. Although the flow rates can start to decrease during exercise, the lowest values usually occur 5 to 12 minutes after 6 to 8 minutes of vigorous exercise.[13] It is well documented that EIB is inhibited by inhaling fully humidified air at 37°C and the primary stimulus to EIB is most likely water lost by evaporation, in humidifying large volumes of air during exercise.[13] The evaporation of water is associated with heat loss and dehydration of the airway surface liquid (ASL). The ASL is 5 to 7 μm in depth; over the first 10 generations of airways, its total volume is estimated to be less than 1 mL.[14] There are 2 major theories for the mechanism whereby respiratory water loss causes bronchoconstriction. One theory relates to the thermal effects[15] and the other relates to the osmotic effects of water loss.[13,14] The thermal theory proposes that the increased ventilation during exercise causes airway cooling and vasoconstriction that is followed by rapid rewarming and a reactive hyperemia of the bronchial mucosal vasculature at the cessation of exercise. These vascular events cause the airways to narrow. The theory does not encompass bronchial smooth muscle or mediator release.[15] The osmotic theory proposes that the water lost by the increased ventilation of exercise transiently increases the osmolarity of the airway surface and possibly the submucosa.[13,14] This hyperosmolarity, in turn, triggers the release of mediators, such as PGs, LTs; histamine from inflammatory cells, such as mast cells and eosinophils; and possibly neuropeptides from sensory nerves in the airways.[16–19] These mediators can cause the airways to narrow by contraction of bronchial smooth muscle.[14]

The documentation of EIB, under conditions of breathing hot dry air, demonstrates that airway cooling is not a prerequisite for EIB.[20] Thus, although the vascular events may play an important role when exercise is performed in low-temperature conditions, these events become less relevant when exercise is performed in moderate- to high-temperature conditions. The importance of increased ventilation, rather than the metabolic effects of exercise, in provoking EIB has been confirmed by studies showing similar results with eucapnic voluntary hyperpnea (EVH).[21] Moreover, the release of mediators has been demonstrated in vivo following inhalation of the osmotically active substance mannitol as well as in vitro.[16,18,22] The protective effect of the mast cell stabilizing agent sodium cromoglycate on challenge by exercise and mannitol supports mediator release from mast cells as an important factor in provoking EIB.[23,24] Further, LT antagonists, such as montelukast, significantly attenuate EIB, whereas histamine seems to have a subordinate role with conflicting results using antihistamines.[25–27]

REFRACTORINESS WITH REPEATED CHALLENGES

McNeill and colleagues[28] were the first to describe refractoriness to repeated exercise challenges, and Edmunds and colleagues[29] were the first to study its duration. Edmunds and colleagues performed a repeated exercise challenge in 8 patients and looked at the duration of the refractory period and the effect of the workload on the degree of refractoriness. The degree of refractoriness varied between the patients, and the duration of the refractory period varied from 1 to 2 hours (**Fig. 2**). The more intense the exercise during the first challenge, the more refractory the patients were to the second challenge.

A refractory period occurs not only after exercise challenge but also after other indirect challenges, such as EVH,[30,31] hypertonic saline,[32] adenosine,[33] ultrasonically nebulized distilled water,[34] and mannitol.[35,36] All these indirect challenges are associated with the release of mediators, all are inhibited by premedication with sodium cromoglycate, and all are thought to induce refractoriness via a similar pathway.[37] EVH is a good surrogate for an exercise challenge producing a similar reduction in lung function and a similar degree of refractoriness.[38] Cross-refractoriness occurs between exercise and EVH,[39] between exercise and hypertonic saline,[40] and between exercise and adenosine 5′-monophoshate.[41] The findings of cross-refractoriness between the different indirect challenges support the concept that they share similar mechanisms. Initial mast cell mediator release is common to all of these challenges.

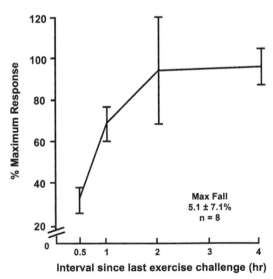

Fig. 2. The duration of refractoriness. Eight patients performed a second running exercise after the specified interval of time. The shorter the time between tests, the less the response on the second test. By 4 hours, the initial response was reestablished. (*From* Edmunds AT, Tooley M, Godfrey S. The refractory period after exercise-induced asthma: its duration and relation to the severity of exercise. Am Rev Respir Dis 1978;117:247–54; with permission.)

SUGGESTED MECHANISMS OF REFRACTORINESS

The mechanisms that have been proposed to account for refractoriness following exercise include high levels of circulating catecholamines, depletion of mast cell mediators, a decrease in release of sensory neuropeptides, a decreased responsiveness of the smooth muscle, release of a protective mediator in response to the initial challenge, and desensitization and/or downregulation of the receptors for the mediators that cause bronchoconstriction after the initial challenge.

Increased Levels of Catecholamines

One of the initial proposals put forward to account for refractoriness was that higher levels of catecholamines released during the first provocation would be protective during the second challenge. This proposal was not supported by studies measuring levels of epinephrine and norepinephrine after exercise and during the refractory period to exercise challenge.[42,43] Further refractoriness has been reported after EVH and other indirect stimuli that do not involve release of catecholamines.[30]

Depletion of Mast Cell Mediators

Over the years, the assays to identify inflammatory mediators in the blood, sputum, and urine became more sensitive, and mediator release as the cause of EIB became more widely accepted. The identification of the involvement of mediator release in EIB led some investigators to propose that refractoriness might be caused by a depletion of these mediators by the initial challenge, with insufficient concentration of mediators remaining to cause bronchoconstriction a second time. This theory became accepted, but there are only a few studies that have actually investigated the possibility of the depletion of mediators after repeated challenge. Belcher and colleagues[43] studied the release of histamine and catecholamines in plasma and venous blood, respectively, following 2 exercise challenges separated by 60 minutes. No difference in the release of histamine or catecholamines between the first and second challenge was seen even though the subjects were refractory. More recently, the authors reported results on the urinary excretion of LTE_4 and PGD_2 following 2 mannitol challenges, 90 minutes apart.[35] The authors found release of both mediators after both challenges, with the subjects who were most refractory having the highest levels of mediators compared with those who were least refractory. Taken together, these two studies do not support depletion of mediators as a cause of refractoriness, and there are no reports of observations of decreased release during the refractory period.

Decreased Release of Sensory Neuropeptides

Evidence to support EIB being mediated by neuropeptides comes from the inhibitory effect of a neurokinin $(NK)_1$ receptor antagonist.[44] There are, however, conflicting data from a study of the effect of a nonselective NK_1/NK_2 receptor antagonist showing no effect on the bronchoconstriction following hypertonic saline.[45] Further, in addition to their well-known effects on mast cells, sodium cromoglycate and nedocromil sodium also have an inhibitory effect on sensory nerves.[46] Other evidence comes from the finding that the release of LTs and NKA (an NK_1/NK_2 receptor agonist) were strongly associated, raising the possibility that the cysteinyl leukotrienes (CysLTs) activated the sensory nerves.[47] This association, however, could also be an effect of the LTs and NKA being released in parallel or that activation of sensory nerves induces the release of mediators from mast cells. The sensory nerves are also activated by increases in osmolarity.[17]

The data to support the depletion of sensory neuropeptides in the development of refractoriness come from the finding that there is cross-refractoriness between sodium metabisulfite, a neurally mediated challenge, and exercise.[48] However, metabisulfite challenge may also be associated with the release of leukotrienes because the CysLT$_1$ antagonist zafirlukast has been shown to attenuate the response to sodium metabisulphite.[49] The involvement of neuropeptides and sensory nerves in the development of refractoriness needs to be further investigated because, to date, only indirect evidence exists and the literature on the effect of neurokinin antagonism is conflicting.[50]

Decreased Responsiveness of the Airway Smooth Muscle

To test if refractoriness is caused by the airway smooth muscle not being able to contract during the second challenge, various pharmacologic agents that act directly on smooth muscle have been administered during the refractory period. The responsiveness of the smooth muscle to inhalation of histamine and methacholine after exercise challenge[51–53] and methacholine after mannitol challenge has been reported as unchanged in subjects who are refractory.[36] A decreased responsiveness to histamine has been documented only after paired, but not single, exercise provocation.[54] Thus, it seems unlikely that refractoriness to EIB can be accounted for by a general decreased responsiveness of the airway smooth muscle itself. Although the muscle may remain responsive to histamine, this mediator does not play a prominent role in sustaining EIB.[27]

Tachyphylaxis of the muscle may occur in response to other mediators of EIB. For example, it is well recognized that tachyphylaxis occurs with repeated inhalation of LTD$_4$ and cross-tachyphylaxis occurs between exercise challenge and LTD$_4$ challenge (**Fig. 3**).[55] One of the original observations on tachyphylaxis involved the inhalation of PGF$_{2\alpha}$ and led to a proposal of a secondary protective mechanism. Fish and colleagues[56] demonstrated that when PGF$_{2\alpha}$ was inhaled, it induced bronchoconstriction; but if the inhalation was continued with higher doses, there was a return to baseline lung function. It was not clear if this tachyphylaxis was an expression of decreased responsiveness of the muscle, by downregulation of the receptor, or caused by the release of a protective substance. Yet another possibility is that PGF2α at the higher concentration, because of its relative lack of receptor specificity, would have also had an effect on other PG receptors, such as the bronchodilating PGE$_2$ receptors EP$_2$ and EP$_4$. It seemed necessary for PGF$_{2\alpha}$ to be the initial stimulus, but the subsequent response was not specific to PGF$_{2\alpha}$ because there was also a reduction in responsiveness to histamine (**Fig. 4**).[56] The investigators suggested that there may be a secondary protective mechanism initiated by PGF$_{2\alpha}$. Hyperventilation has been shown to induce the release of bronchodilating PGE$_2$ and PGI$_2$, lending support to the idea of a secondary protective mechanism involving PGs.[57]

Release of Protective PGs

The release of a protective PG would seem to be the best argued mechanism for refractoriness to date. The proposal of a protective mediator initially made by Fish and colleagues[56] was revisited by others who studied the effect of pretreatment with the cyclooxygenase (COX) inhibitors, thereby blocking the production of prostanoids, such as PGs, prostacyclin, and thromboxane. The effect of the COX inhibitor indomethacin has been studied extensively on refractoriness to exercise, EVH, and inhaled water aerosol (**Fig. 5**).[34,58–60] The findings that indomethacin abolished refractoriness to these 3 challenges, yet had no effect on the response to the initial challenge, strongly support the role of PGs in the development of refractoriness.

The early studies involved an initial exercise breathing hot humid air followed by a second exercise challenge breathing dry air.[61,62] EIB was inhibited by the hot humid

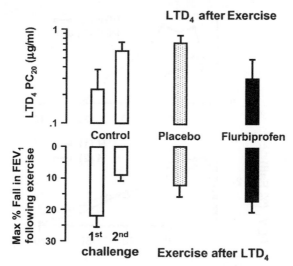

Fig. 3. Cross-refractoriness between exercise and LTD_4. (*Upper panel*) The mean (%SEM) PC_{20} LTD_4 for two LTD_4 challenges separated by 1 hour and for an LTD_4 challenge 1 hour after exercise during treatment with either placebo or flurbiprofen (50 mg/d for 3 days). LTD_4 tachyphylaxis occurred in control subjects (*open bars*). LTD_4 tachyphylaxis also occurred after exercise during placebo (*dotted bars*), but the effect was significantly attenuated ($P = .027$) during flurbiprofen treatment (*solid bars*). (*Lower panel*) The mean (SEM) percentage decrease in FEV_1 after 2 exercise challenges separated by 1 hour and for exercise 1 hour after LTD_4 challenge during treatment with either placebo or flurbiprofen. Exercise refractoriness occurred after LTD_4 challenge during placebo treatment (*dotted bars*), but the effect was significantly attenuated ($P = .026$) during flurbiprofen treatment (*solid bars*). (*From* Manning PJ, Watson RM, O'Byrne PM. Exercise-induced refractoriness in asthmatic subjects involves leukotriene and prostaglandin interdependent mechanisms. Am Rev Respir Dis 1993;148:950–4; with permission.)

air, but tolerance, to a similar degree as refractoriness, was observed to the second exercise with dry air.[61,62] These studies were important because they demonstrated that EIB per se was not required for the development of tolerance to the second exercise. Further, the tolerance to the second exercise was abolished by pretreatment with indomethacin.[60] This finding suggests that protective PGs were induced by the initial exercise challenge, even in the absence of EIB (**Fig. 6**).[60] It also suggests that PGs play no role in the inhibition of EIB by hot humid air because no bronchoconstriction occurred during indomethacin treatment. The inhibitory effect of indomethacin on refractoriness, however, makes the release of a protective PG following initial challenge seem a likely mechanism. There is one major caveat, however, in that severe EIB has been reported when breathing dry air 20 minutes after an initial challenge with hot humid air when EIB was prevented.[63,64] Although these two studies were not designed to include the effect of indomethacin, the findings are markedly at odds with those described earlier.

Further support for a protective PG came from a later study in which the effect of repeated exercise and LTD_4 challenge were investigated as well as the effect of LTD_4 preceding or following exercise challenge.[55] The investigators used the COX inhibitor flurbiprofen to study its effect on the refractory period (see **Fig. 3**). Their findings suggest that LTs induce release of a protective PG. By contrast, there is currently no evidence for a role of histamine in the release of protective mediators.

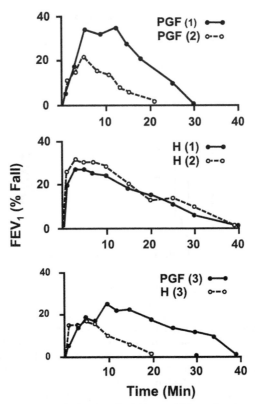

Fig. 4. The effect of repeated inhalation of PGF2α and histamine in patients with asthma. Percent change in FEV$_1$ after administration of different agonist combinations in a representative subject. Panels, from top to bottom, illustrate the response to first (PGF1) and second (PGF2) challenge with PGF$_{2\alpha}$, response to first (H1) and second (H2) challenge with histamine, and response to challenge with PGF$_{2\alpha}$ (PGF3) followed by histamine (H3). Tachyphylaxis to the second challenge with PGF$_{2\alpha}$ was seen. Also a decreased response to histamine was seen following challenge with PGF$_{2\alpha}$. (*From* Fish JE, Jameson LS, Albright A, et al. Modulation of the bronchomotor effects of chemical mediators by prostaglandin F2 alpha in asthmatic subjects. Am Rev Respir Dis 1984;130:571–4; with permission.)

For example, histamine H$_2$-receptor antagonists neither affect the airway response to exercise nor the refractoriness induced with repeated challenges.[65,66] However, the possible role of the more recently discovered H$_3$ and H$_4$ receptors remains to be studied.

This protective PG was considered likely to be PGE$_2$, which had been shown to reduce both the duration and severity of bronchoconstriction following exercise challenge.[67] Inhalation of PGE$_2$ does not alter the airway response to methacholine, suggesting it does not act as a functional antagonist.[67,68] PGE$_2$ may work through mast cells, neural pathways, or via modulation of receptors or downstream intracellular signaling molecules. PGE$_2$ is thought to be produced by the airway smooth muscle cells[69] and the epithelium.[70] An increase in osmolarity is also a stimulus for the release of PGE$_2$.[71] PGE$_2$ also reduces the airway response to metabisulfite. This finding, together with the data supporting a role for leukotrienes in metabisulphite-induced bronchoconstriction, is in keeping with the concept of interdependence between LTs and PGs in the development of refractoriness.

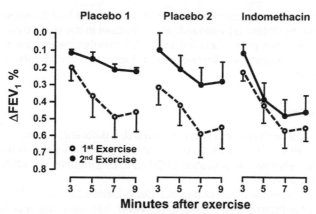

Fig. 5. The effect of indomethacin on the refractory period Change in FEV₁ after exercise on the 2 placebo days. The EIB was similar on the 1st exercise challenge on each test day (*open circles*). Refractoriness occurred after exercise on the 2 placebo days but not after indomethacin. (*From* O'Byrne PM, Jones GL. The effect of indomethacin on exercise-induced bronchoconstriction and refractoriness after exercise. Am Rev Respir Dis 1986;134:69–72; with permission.)

Many studies have suggested this protective PG to be PGE_2.[55,58–60] Although this is the most studied idea, much remains unclear; is there release of PGE_2? If there is release, how does the PGE_2 act to prevent bronchoconstriction? How long lasting is the effect? The reason for this protective PG not affecting the bronchoconstrictor response to the initial challenge, to any significant extent, may be that the release is

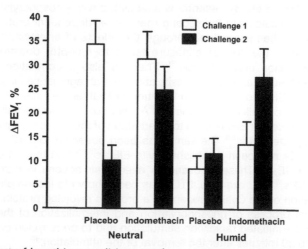

Fig. 6. The effect of breathing conditions on the response to a subsequent challenge performed in thermo neutral conditions. Percentage decrease in FEV₁ (mean ± standard error of the mean) after exercise compared with pre-exercise values. Placebo and indomethacin pretreatments were compared under thermoneutral and warm-humid breathing conditions. Refractoriness was seen during challenge 2 (*closed bars*) independent of the breathing conditions during challenge 1 (*open bars*). The refractoriness was abolished by indomethacin in both situations. (*From* Wilson BA, Bar-Or O, O'Byrne PM. The effects of indomethacin on refractoriness following exercise both with and without a bronchoconstrictor response. Eur Respir J 1994;7:2174–8; with permission.)

delayed compared with the other mediators. It may also be that it needs to be present before the other mediators are released, as is the case in the study by Melillo and colleagues[67] whereby the patient inhaled PGE_2 30 minutes before the challenge. Yet another possibility is that the effectiveness is dependent on interplay with the other released mediators.

WHERE ARE WE NOW?

Since the idea of a protective PG was put forward, 4 different receptors for PGE_2 have been identified, EP_{1-4}. The activation of EP_1 and EP_3 has been shown to induce bronchoconstriction, whereas the activation of EP_2 and EP_4 induces relaxation of the bronchial smooth muscle.[72,73]

Manning and colleagues[55] proposed interdependence between LTs and PGs in the development of refractoriness. This idea, however, has never been proven; and how PGE_2 would exert its effect has not been discussed. Also, that levels of PGE_2 are elevated during the refractory period requires confirmation. Considering the recent findings[35] of a relation between high levels of mediators and a higher degree of refractoriness, the authors propose a new interpretation of how the interplay between LTs and PGs (PGE_2 and PGD_2) takes place: via downregulation of the $CysLT_1$.

From studies investigating G protein–coupled receptors (GPCRs), a common finding is agonist-promoted homologous desensitization.[74] This topic has been extensively investigated with the β_2-adrenergic receptor agonists (β_2 agonist). In relation to EIB, this desensitization to a β_2 agonist manifests as a reduction in the duration of protection against EIB within days of regular use,[75–77] a more prolonged recovery from EIB in response to a β_2 agonist when breakthrough EIB has occurred,[78] and an increase in the severity of EIB at the end of a dosing period.[79] With acute stimulation, this desensitization of the β_2- receptor is associated with phosphorylation of the receptor by GPCR kinases and the second messenger-dependent protein kinase A.[80] The receptors are then internalized through the effects of arrestins.[74] With a more chronic stimulation, the agonist exposure leads to receptor downregulation with decreased expression and synthesis.[80] There is also a correlation between the strength of the stimulus and the desensitization that an agonist can induce.[81]

The various GPCRs do not work in isolation but rather they have been shown to exhibit extensive crosstalk between them.[82] An example of this crosstalk is the activation of the PGE_2 receptor EP_1 leading to a reduction of the bronchodilating function of the β_2-adrenergic receptor.[83] The same has been observed for LTD_4.[84] Release of PGD_2 and CysLTs has been established with EIB[19,85,86] and there are also reports on release of PGE_2.[87] These eicosanoids exert their actions in humans via their respective GPCRs.[88] For example, LTD_4 has been shown to induce phosphorylation and internalization of the $CysLT_1$ receptor, a process involving protein kinase C and arrestins.[89] This process of phosphorylation and internalization of the $CysLT_1$ has been shown to be initiated rapidly on stimulation and to be recycled back to the cell surface in 15 to 20 minutes after the removal of the stimulation.[90]

The early study of EIB showing a relationship between the workload and refractoriness[29] and the more recent study showing higher mediator levels in those who are most refractory[35] is in keeping with receptor desensitization as the mechanism of refractoriness. Also in keeping with receptor desensitization is the prolonged increase (60–120 minutes) in the urinary excretion of LTE_4 and 11β-$PGF_{2\alpha}$ after challenge with exercise, EVH, or mannitol.[19,35,85,86] (The nomenclature of the metabolites of different PGs has recently been revised, and 11β-$PGF_{2\alpha}$ is the new term for the metabolite previously called $9\alpha,11\beta$-PGF_2 by the authors and others.) Further, the timing of induction and cessation of receptor internalization would fit with the duration of the refractory period being up to 2 hours. From the authors' experience,[35,85,86] they have seen that the dynamics of release and the level of mediators vary to a great degree between subjects. These differences between subjects not only help to explain why some subjects are rendered refractory while others are not, but they may also account for the varying duration of the refractory period.[29] When the authors compared the most and least refractory subjects following repeated inhalation of mannitol, they found that the most refractory subjects had significantly higher levels of both LTE_4 and the PGD_2 metabolite 11β-$PGF_{2\alpha}$.[35] The most refractory subjects also had sustained higher levels and did not return to baseline mediator values before the second challenge.

The consistent finding of increased levels of the PGD_2 metabolite 11β-$PGF_{2\alpha}$ during EIB may be relevant in that it may contribute to crosstalk via the thromboxane receptor (TP) receptor leading to desensitization of the $CysLT_1$ (**Fig. 7**). In keeping with this, the effect of indomethacin on refractoriness could be explained by PGs having an important role in the crosstalk between GPCRs to induce increased desensitization of $CysLT_1$ in response to elevated levels of LTs following exercise challenge. When the levels of PGs are decreased, as would be the case with indomethacin pretreatment,

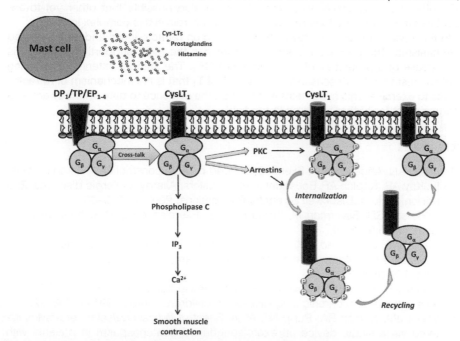

Fig. 7. Desensitization of $CysLT_1$ as a mechanism of refractoriness. With exercise, there is release of cysteinyl leukotrienes from mast cells that stimulate the GPCR $CysLT_1$ causing contraction of the muscle and exercise-induced bronchoconstriction. The PGs generated during the same exercise could, via stimulation of the GPCRs DP_1/EP_{1-4}/TP, lead to crosstalk so that the $CysLT_1$ is desensitized through phosphorylation and internalization. Refractoriness to a second exercise challenge within a short period occurs as a result. When the levels of mediators return to baseline values, the $CysLT_1$ receptors are recycled back to the cell surface and the muscle becomes sensitive to further stimulation. When generation of PGs is inhibited by agents, such as indomethacin and flurbiprofen, then there is limited desensitization of the $CysLT_1$ and, therefore, limited refractoriness. $CysLT_1$, cysteinyl leukotriene receptor$_1$; DP_1, prostaglandin D receptor$_1$; EP_{1-4}, prostaglandin E receptor$_{1-4}$; GPCR, G-protein coupled receptor; TP, thromboxane receptor.

LTs alone would not be able to cause enough phosphorylation to induce refractoriness or at least not as effectively.

Further support for the idea of high levels of CysLTs leading to decreased sensitivity of the same receptor comes from a series of studies of patients with aspirin-intolerant asthma by Lee and coworkers.[91–93] In this peculiar syndrome, following a positive challenge with aspirin causing bronchoconstriction, continued daily administration of aspirin produces a state of refractoriness to aspirin (ie, aspirin desensitization).

If there is a general desensitization of all the receptors of the mediators released during EIB or if there is desensitization only of a specific receptor (eg, the CysLT$_1$) remains to be determined. Also, what receptors are involved with this process either directly or via crosstalk is somewhat speculative, but the PGE$_2$ receptors EP$_{1-4}$, the PGD$_2$ receptors DP$_1$ and TP, and the PGI$_2$ receptor IP are all likely candidates.

There are also experimental data suggesting a possible role for adenosine or ATP. The bronchoconstriction, and the change in volume that may be expected to occur in the ASL during challenge by exercise, EVH, distilled water, hypertonic saline, and mannitol, is likely to lead to the release of ATP.[94] The suggested involvement of adenosine or ATP makes extracellular nucleotide receptors P2Y and the adenosine receptor A2b other possible candidates. It is of course also possible that other yet-to-be-identified mediators and their receptors have a vital role in this complex interplay.

In this review, the authors revisit the literature on refractoriness and its suggested mechanisms. The proposed mechanism that has the most supportive evidence is the release of a protective PG, presumably PGE$_2$. The authors extend this thinking and suggest that it is desensitization of the CysLT$_1$ that is the mechanism of refractoriness to exercise. This hypothesis is based on the evidence to date and may act as a starting point for further research in the field.

REFERENCES

1. Freed AN, Anderson SD. Exercise-induced bronchoconstriction. Human models. In: Kay AB, Kaplan AP, Bousquet J, et al, editors. Allergy & allergic diseases. 2nd edition. Oxford: Blackwell Scientific Publications; 2008. p. 806–20.
2. Anderson SD, Silverman M, Konig P, et al. Exercise-induced asthma. Br J Dis Chest 1975;69:1–39.
3. Cabral AL, Conceicao GM, Fonseca-Guedes CH, et al. Exercise-induced bronchospasm in children: effects of asthma severity. Am J Respir Crit Care Med 1999;159:1819–23.
4. Godfrey S, Springer C, Noviski N, et al. Exercise but not methacholine differentiates asthma from chronic lung disease in children. Thorax 1991;46:488–92.
5. Weiler JM, Nathan RA, Rupp NT, et al. Effect of fluticasone/salmeterol administered via a single device on exercise-induced bronchospasm in patients with persistent asthma. Ann Allergy Asthma Immunol 2005;94:65–72.
6. Anderson SD, Lambert S, Brannan JD, et al. Laboratory protocol for exercise asthma to evaluate salbutamol given by two devices. Med Sci Sports Exerc 2001;33:893.
7. Koh YI, Choi IS, Lim H. Atopy may be related to exercise-induced bronchospasm in asthma. Clin Exp Allergy 2002;32:532–6.
8. Helenius IJ, Tikkanen HO, Haahtela T. Occurrence of exercise induced bronchospasm in elite runners: dependence on atopy and exposure to cold air and pollen. Br J Sports Med 1998;32:125–9.
9. Karjalainen J. Exercise response in 404 young men with asthma: no evidence for a late asthmatic reaction. Thorax 1991;46:100–4.

10. Hofstra WB, Sterk PJ, Neijens HJ, et al. Occurrence of a late response to exercise in asthmatic children: multiple regression approach using time-matched baseline and histamine control days. Eur Respir J 1996;9:1348–55.
11. Schoeffel RE, Anderson SD, Gillam I, et al. Multiple exercise and histamine challenge in asthmatic patients. Thorax 1980;35:164–70.
12. Anderson SD. Exercise-induced asthma: stimulus, mechanism, and management. In: Barnes PJ, Rodger I, Thomson NC, editors. Asthma: basic mechanisms and clinical management. London: Academic Press; 1988. p. 503–22.
13. Anderson SD, Daviskas E. The mechanism of exercise-induced asthma is... J Allergy Clin Immunol 2000;106:453–9.
14. Anderson SD. Is there a unifying hypothesis for exercise-induced asthma? J Allergy Clin Immunol 1984;73:660–5.
15. McFadden ER Jr, Lenner KA, Strohl KP. Postexertional airway rewarming and thermally induced asthma. New insights into pathophysiology and possible pathogenesis. J Clin Invest 1986;78:18–25.
16. Brannan JD, Gulliksson M, Anderson SD, et al. Evidence of mast cell activation and leukotriene release after mannitol inhalation. Eur Respir J 2003;22:491–6.
17. Pisarri TE, Jonson A, Coleridge HM, et al. Intravenous injection of hypertonic NaCl solutions stimulates pulmonary C-fibres in dogs. Am J Physiol 1991;260(5 Pt 2): H1522–30.
18. Gulliksson M, Palmberg L, Nilsson G, et al. Release of prostaglandin D2 and leukotriene C4 in response to hyperosmolar stimulation of mast cells. Allergy 2006;61:1473–9.
19. O'Sullivan S, Roquet A, Dahlen B, et al. Evidence for mast cell activation during exercise-induced bronchoconstriction. Eur Respir J 1998;12:345–50.
20. Anderson SD, Schoeffel RE, Black JL, et al. Airway cooling as the stimulus to exercise-induced asthma–a re-evaluation. Eur J Respir Dis 1985;67:20–30.
21. Rundell KW, Anderson SD, Spiering BA, et al. Field exercise vs laboratory eucapnic voluntary hyperventilation to identify airway hyperresponsiveness in elite cold weather athletes. Chest 2004;125:909–15.
22. Eggleston P, Kagey-Sobotka A, Schleimer R, et al. Interaction between hyperosmolar and IgE-mediated histamine release from basophils and mast cells. Am Rev Respir Dis 1984;130:86.
23. Tullett WM, Tan KM, Wall RT, et al. Dose-response effect of sodium cromoglycate pressurised aerosol in exercise induced asthma. Thorax 1985;40:41–4.
24. Brannan JD, Gulliksson M, Anderson SD, et al. Inhibition of mast cell PGD2 release protects against mannitol-induced airway narrowing. Eur Respir J 2006; 27:944–50.
25. Kemp JP, Dockhorn RJ, Shapiro GG, et al. Montelukast once daily inhibits exercise-induced bronchoconstriction in 6- to 14-year-old children with asthma. J Pediatr 1998;133:424–8.
26. Anderson SD, Brannan JD. Exercise-induced asthma: is there still a case for histamine? J Allergy Clin Immunol 2002;109:771–3.
27. Dahlen B, Roquet A, Inman MD, et al. Influence of zafirlukast and loratadine on exercise-induced bronchoconstriction. J Allergy Clin Immunol 2002;109: 789–93.
28. McNeill RS, Nairn JR, Millar JS, et al. Exercise-induced asthma. Q J Med 1966; 35:55–67.
29. Edmunds AT, Tooley M, Godfrey S. The refractory period after exercise-induced asthma: its duration and relation to the severity of exercise. Am Rev Respir Dis 1978;117:247–54.

30. Bar-Yishay E, Ben-Dov I, Godfrey S. Refractory period after hyperventilation-induced asthma. Am Rev Respir Dis 1983;127:572–4.
31. Argyros GJ, Roach JM, Hurwitz KM, et al. The refractory period after eucapnic voluntary hyperventilation challenge and its effect on challenge technique. Chest 1995;108:419–24.
32. Hawksworth RJ, O'Hickey SP, Lee TH. The effects of indomethacin on the refractory period to hypertonic saline-induced bronchoconstriction. Eur Respir J 1992; 5:963–6.
33. Daxun Z, Rafferty P, Richards R, et al. Airway refractoriness to adenosine 5'-monophosphate after repeated inhalation. J Allergy Clin Immunol 1989;83: 152–8.
34. Mattoli S, Foresi A, Corbo GM, et al. The effect of indomethacin on the refractory period occurring after the inhalation of ultrasonically nebulized distilled water. J Allergy Clin Immunol 1987;79:678–83.
35. Larsson J, Perry CP, Anderson SD, et al. The occurrence of refractoriness and mast cell mediator release following mannitol-induced bronchoconstriction. J Appl Physiol 2011;110:1029–35.
36. Suh DI, Lee JK, Kim JT, et al. Airway refractoriness to inhaled mannitol after repeated challenge. Pediatr Pulmonol 2011;46(10):1007–14.
37. Joos GF, O'Connor B, Anderson SD, et al. Indirect airway challenges. Eur Respir J 2003;21:1050–68.
38. Rosenthal RR, Laube BL, Hood DB, et al. Analysis of refractory period after exercise and eucapnic voluntary hyperventilation challenge. Am Rev Respir Dis 1990; 141:368–72.
39. Ben-Dov I, Gur I, Bar-Yishay E, et al. Refractory period following induced asthma: contributions of exercise and isocapnic hyperventilation. Thorax 1983;38:849–53.
40. Belcher NG, Rees PJ, Clark TJ, et al. A comparison of the refractory periods induced by hypertonic airway challenge and exercise in bronchial asthma. Am Rev Respir Dis 1987;135:822–5.
41. Finnerty J, Polosa R, Holgate S. Repeated exposure of asthmatic airways to inhaled adenosine 5'-monophosphate attenuates bronchoconstriction provoked by exercise. J Allergy Clin Immunol 1990;86:353–9.
42. Dosani R, Van Loon GR, Burki NK. The relationship between exercise-induced asthma and plasma catecholamines. Am Rev Respir Dis 1987;136:973–8.
43. Belcher NG, Murdoch R, Dalton N, et al. Circulating concentrations of histamine, neutrophil chemotactic activity, and catecholamines during the refractory period in exercise-induced asthma. J Allergy Clin Immunol 1988;81:100–10.
44. Ichinose M, Miura M, Yamauchi H, et al. A neurokinin 1-receptor antagonist improves exercise-induced airway narrowing in asthmatic patients. Am J Respir Crit Care Med 1996;153:936.
45. Fahy JV, Wong HH, Geppetti P, et al. Effect of an NK1 receptor antagonist (CP-99,994) on hypertonic saline-induced bronchoconstriction and cough in male asthmatic subjects. Am J Respir Crit Care Med 1995;152:879–84.
46. Dixon CM, Barnes PJ. Bradykinin-induced bronchoconstriction: inhibition by nedocromil sodium and sodium cromoglycate. Br J Clin Pharmacol 1989;27: 831–6.
47. Hallstrand TS, Debley JS, Farin FM, et al. Role of MUC5AC in the pathogenesis of exercise-induced bronchoconstriction. J Allergy Clin Immunol 2007;119: 1092–8.
48. Pavord I, Lazarowicz H, Inchley D, et al. Cross refractoriness between sodium metabisulphite and exercise induced asthma. Thorax 1994;49:245–9.

49. Lazarus SC, Wong HH, Watts MJ, et al. The leukotriene receptor antagonist zafirlukast inhibits sulfur dioxide-induced bronchoconstriction in patients with asthma. Am J Respir Crit Care Med 1997;156:1725–30.
50. Joos GF, Pauwels RA. Tachykinin receptor antagonists: potential in airways diseases. Curr Opin Pharmacol 2001;1:235–41.
51. Hahn AG, Nogrady SG, Tumilty DM, et al. Histamine reactivity during the refractory period after exercise induced asthma. Thorax 1984;39:919–23.
52. Boulet LP, Legris C, Turcotte H. Bronchial responsiveness to histamine after repeated exercise-induced bronchospasm. Respiration 1987;52:237–45.
53. Magnussen H, Reuss G, Jorres R. Airway response to methacholine during exercise induced refractoriness in asthma. Thorax 1986;41:667–70.
54. Carpentiere G, Castello F, Marino S. Airway responsiveness to histamine in patients refractory to repeated exercise. Chest 1988;93:933–6.
55. Manning PJ, Watson RM, O'Byrne PM. Exercise-induced refractoriness in asthmatic subjects involves leukotriene and prostaglandin interdependent mechanisms. Am Rev Respir Dis 1993;148:950–4.
56. Fish JE, Jameson LS, Albright A, et al. Modulation of the bronchomotor effects of chemical mediators by prostaglandin F2 alpha in asthmatic subjects. Am Rev Respir Dis 1984;130:571–4.
57. Ishii Y, Kitamura S. Hyperventilation stimulates the release of prostaglandin I2 and E2 from lung in humans. Prostaglandins 1990;39:685–91.
58. O'Byrne PM, Jones GL. The effect of indomethacin on exercise-induced bronchoconstriction and refractoriness after exercise. Am Rev Respir Dis 1986;134:69–72.
59. Margolskee DJ, Bigby BG, Boushey HA. Indomethacin blocks airway tolerance to repetitive exercise but not to eucapnic hyperpnea in asthmatic subjects. Am Rev Respir Dis 1988;137:842–6.
60. Wilson BA, Bar-Or O, O'Byrne PM. The effects of indomethacin on refractoriness following exercise both with and without a bronchoconstrictor response. Eur Respir J 1994;7:2174–8.
61. Ben-Dov I, Bar-Yishay E, Godfrey S. Refractory period after exercise-induced asthma unexplained by respiratory heat loss. Am Rev Respir Dis 1982;125:530–4.
62. Wilson BA, Bar-Or O, Seed LG. Effects of humid air breathing during arm or treadmill exercise on exercise-induced bronchoconstriction and refractoriness. Am Rev Respir Dis 1990;142:349–52.
63. Hahn AG, Nogrady SG, Burton GR, et al. Absence of refractoriness in asthmatic subjects after exercise with warm, humid inspirate. Thorax 1985;40:418–21.
64. Anderson SD, Daviskas E, Schoeffel RE, et al. Prevention of severe exercise-induced asthma with hot humid air. Lancet 1979;2:629.
65. Nogrady SG, Hahn AG. H2-receptor blockade and exercise-induced asthma. Br J Clin Pharmacol 1984;18:795–7.
66. Manning PJ, Watson R, O'Byrne PM. The effects of H2-receptor antagonists on exercise refractoriness in asthma. J Allergy Clin Immunol 1992;90:125–6.
67. Melillo E, Woolley KL, Manning PJ, et al. Effect of inhaled PGE2 on exercise-induced bronchoconstriction in asthmatic subjects. Am J Respir Crit Care Med 1994;149:1138–41.
68. Pavord ID, Wisniewski A, Mathur R, et al. Effect of inhaled prostaglandin E2 on bronchial reactivity to sodium metabisulphite and methacholine in patients with asthma. Thorax 1991;46:633–7.
69. Delamere F, Holland E, Patel S, et al. Production of PGE2 by bovine cultured airway smooth muscle cells and its inhibition by cyclo-oxygenase inhibitors. Br J Pharmacol 1994;111:983–8.

70. Knight DA, Stewart GA, Lai ML, et al. Epithelium-derived inhibitory prostaglandins modulate human bronchial smooth muscle responses to histamine. Eur J Pharmacol 1995;272:1–11.
71. Hjoberg J, Folkerts G, van Gessel SB, et al. Hyperosmolarity-induced relaxation and prostaglandin release in guinea pig trachea in vitro. Eur J Pharmacol 2000; 398:303–7.
72. Woodward DF, Jones RL, Narumiya S. International union of basic and clinical pharmacology. LXXXIII: classification of prostanoid receptors, updating 15 years of progress. Pharmacol Rev 2011;63(3):471–538.
73. Safholm J, Dahlen SE, Delin I, et al. Prostaglandin E (2) maintains the tone of the guinea pig trachea through a balance between activation of contractile EP (1) receptors and relaxant EP (2) receptors. Br J Pharmacol 2013;168(4):794–806.
74. Perry SJ, Lefkowitz RJ. Arresting developments in heptahelical receptor signaling and regulation. Trends Cell Biol 2002;12:130–8.
75. Simons FE, Gerstner TV, Cheang MS. Tolerance to the bronchoprotective effect of salmeterol in adolescents with exercise-induced asthma using concurrent inhaled glucocorticoid treatment. Pediatrics 1997;99:655–9.
76. Nelson JA, Strauss L, Skowronski M, et al. Effect of long-term salmeterol treatment on exercise-induced asthma. N Engl J Med 1998;339:141–6.
77. Ramage L, Lipworth BJ, Ingram CG, et al. Reduced protection against exercise induced bronchoconstriction after chronic dosing with salmeterol. Respir Med 1994;88:363–8.
78. Haney S, Hancox RJ. Recovery from bronchoconstriction and bronchodilator tolerance. Clin Rev Allergy Immunol 2006;31:181–96.
79. Hancox RJ, Subbarao P, Kamada D, et al. Beta2-agonist tolerance and exercise-induced bronchospasm. Am J Respir Crit Care Med 2002;165:1068–70.
80. McGraw DW, Almoosa KF, Paul RJ, et al. Antithetic regulation by beta-adrenergic receptors of Gq receptor signaling via phospholipase C underlies the airway beta-agonist paradox. J Clin Invest 2003;112:619–26.
81. Kenakin T. Drug efficacy at G protein-coupled receptors. Annu Rev Pharmacol Toxicol 2002;42:349–79.
82. McGraw DW, Elwing JM, Fogel KM, et al. Crosstalk between Gi and Gq/Gs pathways in airway smooth muscle regulates bronchial contractility and relaxation. J Clin Invest 2007;117:1391–8.
83. McGraw DW, Mihlbachler KA, Schwarb MR, et al. Airway smooth muscle prostaglandin-EP1 receptors directly modulate beta2-adrenergic receptors within a unique heterodimeric complex. J Clin Invest 2006;116:1400–9.
84. Rovati GE, Baroffio M, Citro S, et al. Cysteinyl-leukotrienes in the regulation of beta2-adrenoceptor function: an in vitro model of asthma. Respir Res 2006;7:103.
85. Kippelen P, Larsson J, Anderson SD, et al. Effect of sodium cromoglycate on mast cell mediators during hyperpnea in athletes. Med Sci Sports Exerc 2010; 42:1853–60.
86. Kippelen P, Larsson J, Anderson SD, et al. Acute effects of beclomethasone on hyperpnea-induced bronchoconstriction. Med Sci Sports Exerc 2010;42: 273–80.
87. Hallstrand TS, Moody MW, Wurfel MM, et al. Inflammatory basis of exercise-induced bronchoconstriction. Am J Respir Crit Care Med 2005;172:679–86.
88. Boyce JA. Mast cells and eicosanoid mediators: a system of reciprocal paracrine and autocrine regulation. Immunol Rev 2007;217:168–85.
89. Naik S, Billington CK, Pascual RM, et al. Regulation of cysteinyl leukotriene type 1 receptor internalization and signaling. J Biol Chem 2005;280:8722–32.

90. Parhamifar L, Sime W, Yudina Y, et al. Ligand-induced tyrosine phosphorylation of cysteinyl leukotriene receptor 1 triggers internalization and signaling in intestinal epithelial cells. PLoS One 2010;5:e14439.
91. Arm JP, O'Hickey SP, Spur BW, et al. Airway responsiveness to histamine and leukotriene E4 in subjects with aspirin-induced asthma. Am Rev Respir Dis 1989;140:148–53.
92. Nasser SM, Patel M, Bell GS, et al. The effect of aspirin desensitization on urinary leukotriene E4 concentrations in aspirin-sensitive asthma. Am J Respir Crit Care Med 1995;151:1326–30.
93. Sousa AR, Parikh A, Scadding G, et al. Leukotriene-receptor expression on nasal mucosal inflammatory cells in aspirin-sensitive rhinosinusitis. N Engl J Med 2002; 347:1493–9.
94. Tarran R. Regulation of airway surface liquid volume and mucus transport by active ion transport. Proc Am Thorac Soc 2004;1:42–6.

Treatment of Exercise-Induced Bronchoconstriction

Vibeke Backer, MD, DMSci*, Asger Sverrild, MD,
Celeste Porsbjerg, MD, PhD

KEYWORDS

- Exercise • Asthma • Treatment • EIB

KEY POINTS

- Exercise-induced bronchoconstriction (EIB) frequently occurs in youngsters and young adults with asthma.
- Prevention of EIB is possible, either pharmacologically or nonpharmacologically.
- Some treatment modalities are best suited for infrequent EIB.
- Some treatment modalities are best suited for frequent EIB.
- Preventive treatment can be supplemented with short-acting reliever therapy when EIB occurs during exercise.
- Daily use of inhaled corticosteroid (ICS) should be initiated when control of EIB cannot be achieved with nonpharmacologic interventions and reliever therapy alone.
- Although low doses of ICS may have a modest effect on reducing EIB, higher doses are usually very effective in reducing severity of EIB.
- High-intensity warm-up is recommended.

INTRODUCTION

Treatment of exercise-induced bronchoconstriction (EIB) is currently based on the same principles as for asthma treatment in general, that is, a bronchodilating component and an antiinflammatory component. An important challenge in relation to EIB is that adjustment of treatment is based on the frequency of symptoms at rest. According to the Global Initiative for Asthma (GINA) guidelines,[1] those with daily symptoms have moderate persistent asthma and should be treated with inhaled corticosteroids (ICS).[2] Moreover, asthma patients should be able to perform unlimited activity. Currently, there is no entirely clear consensus in international guidelines on how to grade the severity of asthma in persons who complain of frequent asthma during exercise, but have few symptoms at rest. Furthermore, in asthma patients who report

Disclosure Statement: None of the authors has anything to disclose or any conflicts of interest.
Respiratory Research Unit, Department of Respiratory Medicine, Bispebjerg Hospital, University of Copenhagen, Bispebjerg Bakke 23, Copenhagen NV 2400, Denmark
* Corresponding author. Respiratory Research Unit, Department of Respiratory Medicine L, Bispebjerg Hospital, Bispebjerg Bakke 23, 2400 Copenhagen NV, Denmark.
E-mail address: backer@dadlnet.dk

Immunol Allergy Clin N Am 33 (2013) 347–362
http://dx.doi.org/10.1016/j.iac.2013.02.005 immunology.theclinics.com
0889-8561/13/$ – see front matter © 2013 Elsevier Inc. All rights reserved.

EIB-related symptoms, the frequency of symptoms may simply reflect the frequency of physical exercise. Active youngsters and young adults with asthma can experience EIB daily, for example, during sports activities or when cycling as a means of transport. These activities could lead to use of beta$_2$-agonist on a daily basis.[3] The problem is that frequent use of a beta$_2$-agonist is a sign of partly controlled disease, which should logically lead to introduction of ICS treatment. However, tolerance may occur if ICS is prescribed in combination with a long-acting beta$_2$-agonist (LABA) on a daily basis.[4,5] This tolerance manifests itself as a reduction in the duration of the protective effect of a beta$_2$-agonist against EIB and slower recovery of lung function in response to further treatment with a bronchodilator if relief is required after exercise or in an emergency.

EIB is an acute event with transient narrowing of the airways occurring during and particularly after exercise.[6] The symptoms of EIB range from a slight feeling of chest tightness with a small reduction in lung function to severe bronchospasm and a large reduction in FEV$_1$ after exercise. Documenting EIB with a reduction in FEV$_1$ of at least 10% from the pre-exercise values is considered to be specific for asthma, but exercise itself is not a sensitive means of diagnosing asthma.[7,8] Individuals with asthma who develop EIB generally report symptoms such as cough, wheeze, chest tightness, dyspnoea, and fatigue.[6] These symptoms are also frequent in healthy individuals particularly while running, in nonasthmatic elite athletes, individuals who are not physically fit, and sometimes in those with extrathoracic disorders such as vocal cord dysfunction.[9]

EIB is most often a sign of eosinophilic airway inflammation and poor asthma control.[10] The high ventilation required during intense exercise leads to airway narrowing because of the osmotic and thermal consequences of evaporative water loss from the airway surface.[11] The dehydration of the airway surface provides a favorable environment for release of mediators that cause airway smooth muscle contraction with or without edema.[6,12,13] In a minority of individuals, primarily elite athletes, EIB can also develop without underlying eosinophilic airway inflammation[4] and, in this group, probably reflects a different pathogenesis.[5,14]

Another issue is the different inflammation associated with EIB.[15] In most asthma patients the inflammation is due to eosinophils, whereas in elite athletes the inflammation may be due to neutrophils and macrophages.[16–18] In the study in asthmatics by Duong and colleagues,[19] a close association was found between number of sputum eosinophils and fall in FEV$_1$ after exercise when testing general asthma patients (**Fig. 1**). The relative contribution of these different types of inflammation or the precise mechanism for eosinophils in the development of EIB is currently unclear. For example, it is not known if some cases of EIB would benefit from medications targeting inflammatory pathways other than the classical type II pathway.

TREATMENT OF EIB

Short-acting beta$_2$-agonists (SABAs) or LABAs are established as preventive or acute treatment of EIB. For frequent respiratory symptoms, however, bronchodilator as needed might not be sufficient, necessitating the addition of daily therapy with an ICS. Antileukotrienes and mast cell stabilizing drugs, such as sodium cromoglycate and nedocromil sodium, are used either as a single drug or in combination with other drugs. Lastly, omega-3, vitamins, and other nonpharmacologic interventions such as vitamins are frequently used for EIB by elite athletes.[20]

Beta$_2$-agonists

SABAs are the drugs of choice for prophylaxis of EIB and for treatment of bronchoconstriction developed during and after exercise.[3] If taken at least 5 minutes before

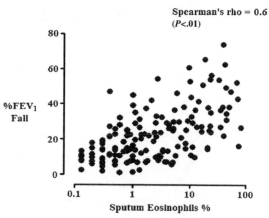

Fig. 1. The severity of EIB expressed as percentage fall in FEV_1 in relation to the percentage of eosinophils in sputum showing an association between sputum cell count and fall in FEV_1 after exercise. All visits were included in analysis. (*Data from* Duong M, Subbarao P, Adelroth E, et al. Sputum eosinophils and the response of exercise-induced bronchoconstriction to corticosteroid in asthma. Chest 2008;133:404–11.)

exercise,[21] a SABA reduces the post-exercise fall in lung function by 70%.[3] In a study by Küpper and colleagues,[22] a mean standard deviation (SD) increase in FEV_1 of 5% ± 6 after a SABA and decrease of 31% ± 11 after placebo was documented in response to a standardized exercise challenge in a group of asthmatic patients (**Fig. 2**). These findings indicate that bronchodilator therapy not only prevents development of EIB but also Induces an increase in FEV_1 in an asthmatic subject when used immediately before physical activity.

SABAs are frequently used as monotherapy, for prophylaxis and treatment of EIB, because of lack of awareness of asthma severity by both the patient and the doctor.[23] In a recent asthma survey as many as 22% of subjects reported taking a beta$_2$-agonist only before exercise, even though they were exercising every day.[10] This figure was even higher (38%) in cases with doctor-diagnosed EIB, indicating that a substantial number of asthma patients frequently use a beta$_2$-agonist before exercise. Furthermore, 19% and 47% used a beta$_2$-agonist as rescue therapy during and after exercise, respectively (**Fig. 3**).[10] These percentages indicate a substantial overuse of beta$_2$-agonist arising from asthma patients using the medication routinely pre-exercise, either from anxiety about an EIB attack to come, or simply because their asthma is undertreated. Daily use of a SABA usually indicates poor asthma control and warrants reassessment of asthma treatment.

The onset of action depends on the beta$_2$-agonist chosen: the onset of action of formoterol, an LABA is as rapid as that of a SABA, whereas salmeterol, another LABA, has a slower onset of action than salbutamol/albuterol.[24] However, the total period of protection is similar for both formoterol and salmeterol. In the study by Richter and colleagues,[25] equipotent doses of formoterol, salmeterol, and terbutaline prevented EIB with a comparable effect, even though the time to the maximal bronchodilating effect was different.

DEVELOPMENT OF TOLERANCE

Regular use of SABAs may lead to development of tolerance to their therapeutic effects. Tolerance to the bronchodilator effects of a beta$_2$-agonist develops rapidly after

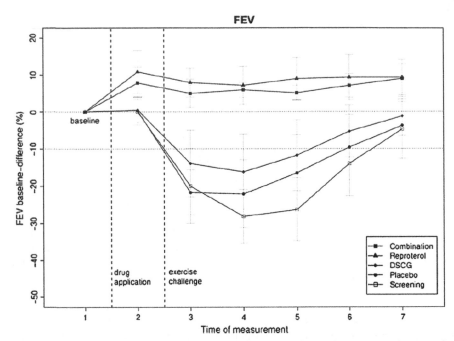

Fig. 2. Mean values (SD) for FEV_1 values for all subjects after sodium cromoglycate, after beta$_2$-agonist, and after both drugs were taken together. The figure illustrates a significantly better effect of beta$_2$-agonist compared with cromoglycate, but no additional effect when both drugs are taken together. (*Reproduced from* Kupper T, Goebbels K, Kennes LN, et al. Cromoglycate, reproterol, or both-what's best for exercise-induced asthma? Sleep Breath 2012;16:1229–35.)

only a few doses, and tolerance to the protective effect occurs irrespective of concomitant use with ICS. The former is of importance in respect of treatment of acute asthma, whereas the latter may lead to inability to prevent EIB.[26–29] Several studies have shown development of tolerance after regular use of LABA, demonstrated by a reduction in the duration of the protective effect against EIB over time.[30–33] Haney and Hancox[29] demonstrated that after 8 days of treatment with formoterol the effect of a SABA was reduced when given after an acute attack of bronchoconstriction, and the area under the salbutamol FEV_1 response curve was significantly reduced from 205 ± 63 SD %.time to 107 ± 53 SD $P<.001$ following treatment (**Fig. 4**).[29] These findings are supported by a study by Elers J and colleagues,[27] who showed a reduction in response of FEV_1 to beta$_2$-agonist of 0.5 L in absolute values compared with the response before LABA treatment. However, beta$_2$-agonist–induced tolerance is not found by all researchers,[34–36] although this could be due to study design. The decrease in duration of protection by a beta$_2$-agonist[30–33] might result in increased use of beta$_2$-agonist and a higher risk of side effects, such as tremor and palpitations, which are dose related, and maybe drug specific. LABA should never be used as monotherapy in asthma because of the potential risk of increased morbidity and mortality during an exacerbation,[37] although not shown by all.[38,39]

There is very little clinical evidence that use of a SABA leads to failure to respond to emergency asthma treatment,[26,40,41] whereas in the case of acute admission higher doses of beta$_2$-agonists are used.

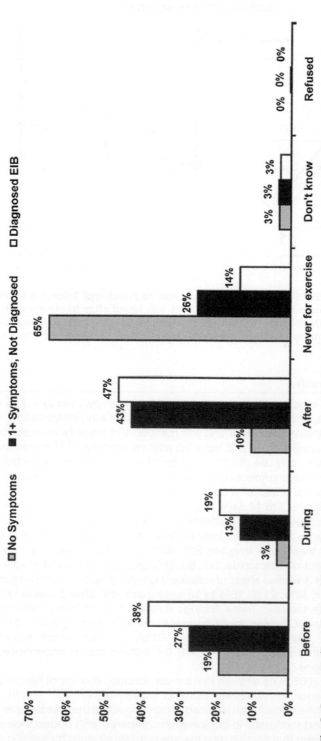

Fig. 3. Rescue medication use while exercising. The association is between the diagnosis of EIB and the use of bronchodilator before, during, or after exercise. Patients who knew that their shortness of breath developed during exercise used SABA more frequently than persons without this knowledge. (*Reproduced from* Parsons JP, Craig TJ, Stoloff SW, et al. Impact of exercise-related respiratory symptoms in adults with asthma: exercise-induced bronchospasm landmark national survey. Allergy Asthma Proc 2011;32:431–7.)

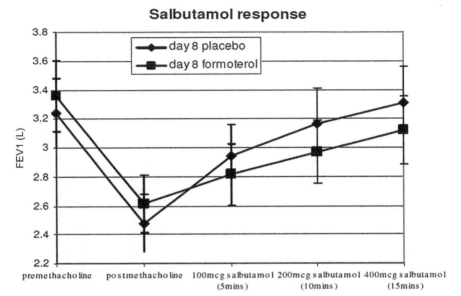

Fig. 4. The mean ± SE FEV₁ Liters (y axis) in response to salbutamol following a methacholine challenge. A reduced response to salbutamol was found after treatment with formoterol after 8 days. (*Reproduced from* Haney S, Hancox RJ. Tolerance to bronchodilation during treatment with long-acting beta-agonists, a randomised controlled trial. Respir Res 2005;6:107.)

Inhaled Corticosteroids

ICS are the most effective inhaled antiinflammatory therapy available. ICS reduce asthma symptoms, improve lung function, decrease airway inflammation, reduce airway hyperresponsiveness (AHR) and the number and severity of exacerbations, thereby improving quality of life and reducing asthma mortality.[42,43] According to international guidelines, daily use of ICS should be initiated when asthma control cannot be achieved with nonpharmacologic interventions and reliever therapy alone. Although the beneficial effect of a single dose of ICS on EIB has been found,[44,45] the effect increases over 7 to 14 days, and the maximum effect can be expected after at least 8 weeks of therapy. Most guidelines suggest use of low-dose ICS. Although this approach may be adequate to treat asthma patients without EIB, it is likely to be inadequate for those with frequent EIB. Subbarao and colleagues[46] showed a dose-response effect of ciclesonide, (40, 80, 160, and 320 μg daily) ICS as well as a period (1 week and 3 weeks) effect of treatment on EIB (**Fig. 5**). The maximum fall in FEV₁ changed from 30%, 21%, 16% to 13%, respectively, after 3 weeks on 320 μg daily of ciclesonide therapy. These findings suggest that, in those with persistent EIB, stepping up the ICS dose might be preferable to adding another type of antiasthma treatment; this is in contrast to the GINA guideline, which recommends add-on therapy with inhaled LABAs to ICS for asthma that is uncontrolled when treated with ICS alone.

In a review from 2005, data showed that the combination therapy of fluticasone and salmeterol is superior to fluticasone alone in preventing EIB.[47,48] Another study showed better asthma control with reduced symptoms when the disease was treated with budesonide and formoterol in combination compared with budesonide alone.[49] These findings suggest that combination therapy is a safe strategy for treating asthma,

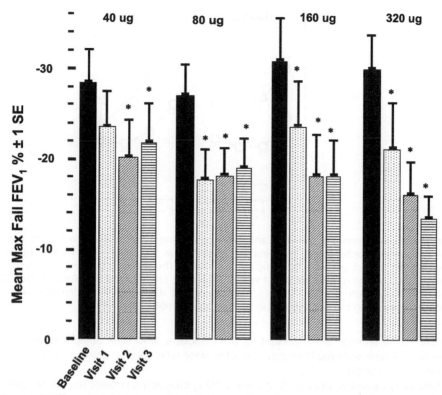

Fig. 5. Effect of increasing doses of inhaled steroid on the percentage fall in FEV$_1$ after exercise at baseline and at Visit 1 after 1 week, at Visit 2 after 2 weeks, and at Visit 3 after 3 weeks treatment with ciclesonide given by inhalation once daily in the evening. The higher doses of ICS – the lower fall in FEV$_1$ after exercise. (*Reproduced from* Subbarao P, Duong M, Adelroth E, et al. Effect of ciclesonide dose and duration of therapy on exercise-induced bronchoconstriction in patients with asthma. J Allergy Clin Immunol 2006;117:1008–13.)

but a problem being that the doses of ICS used might be too low to be effective in preventing EIB in all subjects.

Young adults with EIB, who do recreational sports of less than 10 hours per week, may have classic eosinophilic asthma and accordingly have good sensitivity to treatment with ICS. These asthma patients should, in accordance with the guidelines, be treated with daily doses of ICS either alone or in combination with LABA or an antileukotriene, although the use of ICS does not prevent the development of tolerance to beta$_2$-agnoists.[31,50] In the study by Duong and colleagues,[19] it was shown that although low dose (400 and 800 µg daily) of ICS reduced severity EIB, it did not do so increasingly over time. This reduction in EIB severity at a low dose was independent of the cellular content of sputum being eosinophilic or neutrophilic (**Fig. 6**, left hand panel). However, when treating with the higher doses of ICS (160 or 320 µg daily) (see **Fig. 6**, right hand panel), a significant and continuous reduction was observed in the percentage fall in FEV$_1$ after exercise. These findings were even more pronounced in those with sputum eosinophilia compared with those with sputum neutrophilia, with a mean improvement in fall in FEV$_1$ of 24% versus 14%, *P*<.01. These findings suggest that stepping up the dose of ICS rather than adding on a LABA will lead to better control of EIB, and tolerance does not develop to ICS as it does to a

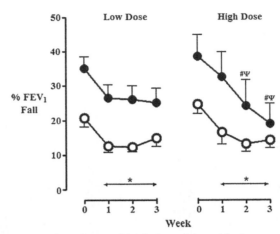

Fig. 6. Exercise response to low-dose and high-dose ciclesonide therapy according to baseline sputum eosinophil count. The data are presented as the mean ± SE noneosinophilic group (*open circles*), eosinophilic group (*closed circles*). The group of patients with eosinophilic asthma achieved a better effect with ICS on their EIB. (*Reproduced from* Duong M, Subbarao P, Adelroth E, et al. Sputum eosinophils and the response of exercise-induced bronchoconstriction to corticosteroid in asthma. Chest 2008;133:404–11.)

LABA. These findings are important for the clinicians, who seek objective measurements in clinical settings, to ensure that otherwise well- treated asthma patients can exercise without EIB.

Elite athletes and young adults who are training daily at the subelite level may have a different inflammatory phenotype.[51] In elite athletes, the airway inflammation may not be of the eosinophilic type and ICS may be less effective, as has been found in skiers.[52] In the daily clinical setting, both sports-active patients and elite athletes need treatment with ICS. The dose of ICS should be titrated so that exercise is possible without symptoms of asthma and without EIB; this may involve up or down titration of steroid dose with down titration being performed in accordance with response to an asthma challenge test, and not symptoms alone.[19,52] Down titration of ICS following high doses of ICS is an issue by itself, and very few, if any, have reported findings in this area of interest.[52] One way to assess asthma control in elite athletes could be by measuring AHR to indirect stimuli and adjusting doses until AHR is obliterated entirely.

Antileukotrienes

Antileukotrienes have antiinflammatory actions and prevent bronchoconstriction over time[53] and include the leukotriene synthesis inhibitors (eg, zileuton) and receptor antagonists (eg, montelukast). They do not have an acute bronchodilator effect and cannot reverse EIB. When compared with albuterol, montelukast was not as effective if taken immediately before exercise.[54] In addition, montelukast is less effective than low-dose ICS.[55] In contrast to beta$_2$-agonists however, daily use of montelukast does not lead to development of tolerance over time (**Fig. 7**).[33,56,57]

Antileukotrienes are given orally and are administered once daily for montelukast and twice daily for zileuton.[58] Although the reduction in the mean overall symptom intensity score was significantly better with zileuton compared with montelukast [−5.0 ± 2.1 (4.6–5.4) vs −4.2 ± 2.3 (3.8–4.7) ($P<.05$)], the same reduction was not observed for the individual symptom scores. Although these findings suggest that

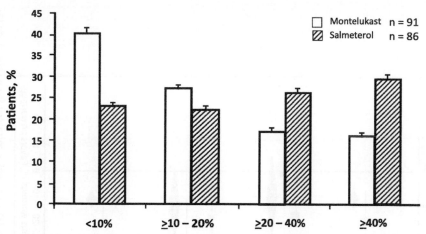

Fig. 7. The percentage fall in FEV_1 after exercise 8 weeks after daily treatment with salmeterol and montelukast. The bronchoprotective effect of montelukast was retained after 8 weeks with the most of the subjects having less than 10% fall in FEV_1 after exercise, whereas the protective effect of salmeterol decreased so that there were fewer subjects who had a less than 10% fall in FEV_1 after exercise and more with a fall greater than 40% compared with montelukast. (*Reproduced from* Edelman JM, Turpin JA, Bronsky EA, et al. Oral montelukast compared with inhaled salmeterol to prevent exercise-induced bronchoconstriction. A randomized, double-blind trial. Exercise Study Group. Ann Intern Med 2000;132:97–104.)

zileuton might be superior, serious side effects have led to removal of the drug from the lists of approved drugs for sport. Montelukast is also used as an add-on therapy when asthma is uncontrolled with medium-dose ICS alone.[59] Studies have reported a reduced fall in FEV_1 and a reduced period of bronchoconstriction after exercise when treated with montelukast, compared with placebo in asthmatic nonsmokers[60] as well as asthma patients in general.[61] Montelukast is effective when given as a single dose 2 hours before exercise[61–63] and would be a satisfactory choice as monotherapy in individuals with EIB who exercise a couple of times per week. However, the effect of montelukast is heterogeneous, being effective in some, and without effect in others.

Mast Cell Stabilizers

The airway narrowing from EIB is thought to be a consequence of the release of inflammatory mediators from the mast cell in response to an increase in osmolarity.[64,65] The use of mast cell stabilizer treatment, such as nedocromil and cromoglycate, should theoretically have a beneficial effect on EIB. These mast cell stabilizers have been shown to be superior to placebo in pharmaceutical studies.[66] They also have an excellent safety profile, a dose-related response, which could be useful in EIB but are limited by their short duration of protection. Studies have shown that use of a SABA is superior to nedocromil.[67] In the study by Küpper and colleagues,[22] the effect of cromoglycate was less than that found after use of a beta$_2$-agonist. The average fall in FEV_1 after placebo was 25% and only 15% after treatment with cromoglycate ($P<.01$), whereas an increase in FEV_1 was found after beta$_2$-agonist (see **Fig. 2**). No additional effect was found when combining the 2 treatments. Studies have shown a relatively lower protection against EIB when using mast cell stabilizer when compared with ICS, although the reason for this is unclear.[68] Although these mast

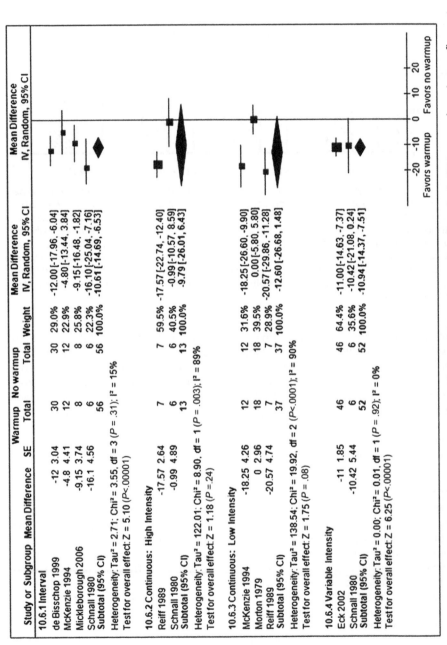

Fig. 8. Warm-up versus no warm-up in pre-exercise treatment of EIB: maximum percentage decrease in FEV_1 or peak expiratory flow rate. A meta-analysis showed a positive effect of warm-up on the development of EIB. (*Reproduced from* Stickland MK, Rowe BH, Spooner CH, et al. Effect of warm-up exercise on exercise-induced bronchoconstriction. Med Sci Sports Exerc 2012;44:383–91.)

cell stabilizers are effective against EIB, they are seldom used nowadays for treatment of asthma in general.

Omega-3, Fish Oil, and Vitamin

Several studies have examined the effect of fish oil in treating mild exercise–induced asthma and especially in some elite athletes in whom it has been shown that the fall in FEV1 after exercise is reduced after 3 weeks' intake of fish oil capsules.[69–73] Fish oil is rich in omega-3 fatty acids, which are thought to compete with proinflammatory mediators and cytokines in reducing EIB. Although both montelukast and fish oils have a protective effect on EIB, the combination of the 2 drugs did not have an additive effect,[69] suggesting that they work through the same pathways.[74–76] In some patients with signs of exercise-induced asthma, the use of vitamin C might have a significant effect[74] and more reactivity to exercise was found in children with low levels of vitamin D.[77] It is not known however whether treatment with vitamin D would decrease the severity of EIB as no intervention studies have been performed.

NONPHARMACOLOGIC THERAPY

There is evidence that physical warm-up reduces EIB in asthmatic athletes. The most consistent and effective attenuation of EIB was observed with high-intensity interval and variable intensity pre-exercise warm-ups.[78] In a review including a meta-analysis concerning the same issue by the same research group,[78] these findings were further supported, as shown in **Fig. 8**. In conclusion, it seems likely that any form of pre-exercise warm-up is of significant importance for the reduction of EIB among asthmatic individuals. This is important information as most asthma patients have EIB and might well gain from doing pre-exercise warm-up.

Many winter-sport athletes, especially cross-country skiers, wear breathing filters for protection against cold air; few, if any, controlled studies exist in this area.[79,80] Other issues of importance might be the number of environmental particles, where a high concentration of small particles is increasingly being associated with the presence of asthma.[81]

SUMMARY

EIB is the major complaint in asthma, and EIB should be treated in accordance with the general asthma guidelines. Given that EIB may relate to mechanisms other than the TH2 pathway in asthma, especially in elite athletes, it is possible that other types of medication could target EIB more specifically. An open question is whether EIB represents mild asthma that is revealed by intense physical exercise or whether different mechanisms are important in the more severe cases of EIB with large fall in FEV_1 as well as asthma symptoms. SABA as a preventer and reliever medication may be sufficient for most cases of EIB, but daily use of ICS should be initiated when asthma control cannot be achieved with nonpharmacologic interventions and reliever therapy alone. Add-on therapy with antileukotrienes, mast cell stabilizers, or omega-3 as well as vitamins should be considered, as they all reduce the fall in FEV_1 after exercise. However, none of these drugs can be used acutely when asthma develops during exercise and none can be used as reliever therapy in post-exercise EIB. Asthma symptoms with frequent use of SABA (>2 times per week) indicate the need to review asthma management. As frequent or daily use of LABA can lead to development of tolerance, ICS are the drug of choice. The dose of ICS should be increased from a low to high dose in cases with persistent EIB. From clinical experience, patients with frequent EIB, such as elite athletes with asthma, often need high doses of ICS to achieve sufficient control.

REFERENCES

1. Bousquet J. Global initiative for asthma (GINA) and its objectives. Clin Exp Allergy 2000;30(Suppl 1):2–5.
2. Bousquet J, Annesi-Maesano I, Carat F, et al. Characteristics of intermittent and persistent allergic rhinitis: DREAMS study group. Clin Exp Allergy 2005;35: 728–32.
3. Anderson SD, Caillaud C, Brannan JD. Beta2-agonist and exercise-induced asthma. Clin Rev Allergy Immunol 2006;31:163–80.
4. Backer V, Rasmussen LM. Exercise-induced asthma symptoms and nighttime asthma: are they similar to ahr? J Allergy (Cairo) 2009;2009:378245.
5. Pedersen L, Lund TK, Molgaard E, et al. The acute effect of swimming on airway inflammation in adolescent elite swimmers. J Allergy Clin Immunol 2009;123: 502–4.
6. Parsons JP, Mastronarde JG. Exercise-induced bronchoconstriction in athletes. Chest 2005;128:3966–74.
7. Eliasson AH, Phillips YY, Rajagopal KR, et al. Sensitivity and specificity of bronchial provocation testing. An evaluation of four techniques in exercise-induced bronchospasm. Chest 1992;102:347–55.
8. Backer V, Bach-Mortensen N, Becker U, et al. The effect of astemizole on bronchial hyperresponsiveness and exercise-induced asthma in children. Allergy 1989;44:209–13.
9. Doshi DR, Weinberger MM. Long-term outcome of vocal cord dysfunction. Ann Allergy Asthma Immunol 2006;96:794–9.
10. Parsons JP, Craig TJ, Stoloff SW, et al. Impact of exercise-related respiratory symptoms in adults with asthma: exercise-induced bronchospasm landmark national survey. Allergy Asthma Proc 2011;32:431–7.
11. Evans TM, Rundell KW, Beck KC, et al. Cold air inhalation does not affect the severity of EIB after exercise or eucapnic voluntary hyperventilation. Med Sci Sports Exerc 2005;37:544–9.
12. DiDario AG, Becker JM. Asthma, sports, and death. Allergy Asthma Proc 2005; 26:341–4.
13. Randolph CC. Allergic rhinitis and asthma in the athlete. Allergy Asthma Proc 2006;27:104–9.
14. Pedersen L, Lund TK, Barnes PJ, et al. Airway responsiveness and inflammation in adolescent elite swimmers. J Allergy Clin Immunol 2008;122:322–7, 327.e1.
15. Jayaram L, Pizzichini MM, Cook RJ, et al. Determining asthma treatment by monitoring sputum cell counts: effect on exacerbations. Eur Respir J 2006;27:483–94.
16. Sue-Chu M, Brannan JD, Anderson SD, et al. Airway hyperresponsiveness to methacholine, adenosine 5-monophosphate, mannitol, eucapnic voluntary hyperpnoea and field exercise challenge in elite cross-country skiers. Br J Sports Med 2010;44:827–32.
17. Sue-Chu M, Henriksen AH, Bjermer L. Non-invasive evaluation of lower airway inflammation in hyper-responsive elite cross-country skiers and asthmatics. Respir Med 1999;93:719–25.
18. Sue-Chu M, Larsson L, Moen T, et al. Bronchoscopy and bronchoalveolar lavage findings in cross-country skiers with and without "ski asthma". Eur Respir J 1999; 13:626–32.

19. Duong M, Subbarao P, Adelroth E, et al. Sputum eosinophils and the response of exercise-induced bronchoconstriction to corticosteroid in asthma. Chest 2008; 133:404–11.
20. Heikkinen A, Alaranta A, Helenius I, et al. Dietary supplementation habits and perceptions of supplement use among elite Finnish athletes. Int J Sport Nutr Exerc Metab 2011;21:271–9.
21. Godfrey S, Bar-Yishay E. Exercised-induced asthma revisited. Respir Med 1993; 87:331–44.
22. Kupper T, Goebbels K, Kennes LN, et al. Cromoglycate, reproterol, or both-what's best for exercise-induced asthma? Sleep Breath 2012;16:1229–35.
23. Backer V, Harmsen L, Lund T, et al. A 3-year longitudinal study of asthma quality of life in undiagnosed and diagnosed asthma patients. Int J Tuberc Lung Dis 2007;11:463–9.
24. Anderson SD, Rodwell LT, Du TJ, et al. Duration of protection by inhaled salmeterol in exercise-induced asthma. Chest 1991;100:1254–60.
25. Richter K, Janicki S, Jorres RA, et al. Acute protection against exercise-induced bronchoconstriction by formoterol, salmeterol and terbutaline. Eur Respir J 2002; 19:865–71.
26. Haney S, Hancox RJ. Recovery from bronchoconstriction and bronchodilator tolerance. Clin Rev Allergy Immunol 2006;31:181–96.
27. Elers J, Strandbygaard U, Pedersen L, et al. Daily use of salmeterol causes tolerance to bronchodilation with terbutaline in asthmatic subjects. Open Respir Med J 2010;4:48–50.
28. Haney S, Hancox RJ. Overcoming beta-agonist tolerance: high dose salbutamol and ipratropium bromide. Two randomised controlled trials. Respir Res 2007;8:19.
29. Haney S, Hancox RJ. Tolerance to bronchodilation during treatment with long-acting beta-agonists, a randomised controlled trial. Respir Res 2005;6:107.
30. Ramage L, Lipworth BJ, Ingram CG, et al. Reduced protection against exercise induced bronchoconstriction after chronic dosing with salmeterol. Respir Med 1994;88:363–8.
31. Simons FE, Gerstner TV, Cheang MS. Tolerance to the bronchoprotective effect of salmeterol in adolescents with exercise-induced asthma using concurrent inhaled glucocorticoid treatment. Pediatrics 1997;99:655–9.
32. Nelson JA, Strauss L, Skowronski M, et al. Effect of long-term salmeterol treatment on exercise-induced asthma. N Engl J Med 1998;339:141–6.
33. Edelman JM, Turpin JA, Bronsky EA, et al. Oral montelukast compared with inhaled salmeterol to prevent exercise-induced bronchoconstriction. A randomized, double-blind trial. Exercise Study Group. Ann Intern Med 2000;132:97–104.
34. Pauwels RA, Lofdahl CG, Postma DS, et al. Effect of inhaled formoterol and budesonide on exacerbations of asthma. Formoterol and Corticosteroids Establishing Therapy (FACET) International Study Group. N Engl J Med 1997;337:1405–11.
35. Davis BE, Reid JK, Cockcroft DW. Formoterol thrice weekly does not result in the development of tolerance to bronchoprotection. Can Respir J 2003;10:23–6.
36. Ni CM, Greenstone IR, Ducharme FM. Addition of inhaled long-acting beta2-agonists to inhaled steroids as first line therapy for persistent asthma in steroid-naive adults. Cochrane Database Syst Rev 2005;(2):CD005307.
37. Rodrigo GJ, Moral VP, Marcos LG, et al. Safety of regular use of long-acting beta agonists as monotherapy or added to inhaled corticosteroids in asthma. A systematic review. Pulm Pharmacol Ther 2009;22:9–19.

38. de Vries F, Setakis E, Zhang B, et al. Long-acting {beta}2-agonists in adult asthma and the pattern of risk of death and severe asthma outcomes: a study using the GPRD. Eur Respir J 2010;36:494–502.

39. Lazarus SC, Boushey HA, Fahy JV, et al. Long-acting beta2-agonist monotherapy vs continued therapy with inhaled corticosteroids in patients with persistent asthma: a randomized controlled trial. JAMA 2001;285:2583–93.

40. Hancox RJ, Le Souef PN, Anderson GP, et al. Asthma: time to confront some inconvenient truths. Respirology 2010;15:194–201.

41. Hancox RJ, Taylor DR. Long-acting beta-agonist treatment in patients with persistent asthma already receiving inhaled corticosteroids. BioDrugs 2001;15: 11–24.

42. Jeffery PK, Godfrey RW, Adelroth E, et al. Effects of treatment on airway inflammation and thickening of basement membrane reticular collagen in asthma. A quantitative light and electron microscopic study. Am Rev Respir Dis 1992;145: 890–9.

43. Suissa S, Ernst P, Benayoun S, et al. Low-dose inhaled corticosteroids and the prevention of death from asthma. N Engl J Med 2000;343:332–6.

44. Kippelen P, Larsson J, Anderson SD, et al. Acute effects of beclomethasone on hyperpnea-induced bronchoconstriction. Med Sci Sports Exerc 2010;42:273–80.

45. Driessen JM, Nieland H, van der Palen JA, et al. Effects of a single dose inhaled corticosteroid on the dynamics of airway obstruction after exercise. Pediatr Pulmonol 2011;46:849–56.

46. Subbarao P, Duong M, Adelroth E, et al. Effect of ciclesonide dose and duration of therapy on exercise-induced bronchoconstriction in patients with asthma. J Allergy Clin Immunol 2006;117:1008–13.

47. Weiler JM, Nathan RA, Rupp NT, et al. Effect of fluticasone/salmeterol administered via a single device on exercise-induced bronchospasm in patients with persistent asthma. Ann Allergy Asthma Immunol 2005;94:65–72.

48. Reynolds NA, Lyseng-Williamson KA, Wiseman LR. Inhaled salmeterol/fluticasone propionate: a review of its use in asthma. Drugs 2005;65:1715–34.

49. Noonan M, Rosenwasser LJ, Martin P, et al. Efficacy and safety of budesonide and formoterol in one pressurised metered-dose inhaler in adults and adolescents with moderate to severe asthma: a randomised clinical trial. Drugs 2006; 66:2235–54.

50. Spector S, Tan R. Exercise-induced bronchoconstriction update: therapeutic management. Allergy Asthma Proc 2012;33:7–12.

51. Lotvall J, Akdis CA, Bacharier LB, et al. Asthma endotypes: a new approach to classification of disease entities within the asthma syndrome. J Allergy Clin Immunol 2011;127:355–60.

52. Sue-Chu M, Karjalainen EM, Laitinen A, et al. Placebo-controlled study of inhaled budesonide on indices of airway inflammation in bronchoalveolar lavage fluid and bronchial biopsies in cross-country skiers. Respiration 2000;67:417–25.

53. Leigh R, Vethanayagam D, Yoshida M, et al. Effects of montelukast and budesonide on airway responses and airway inflammation in asthma. Am J Respir Crit Care Med 2002;166:1212–7.

54. Raissy HH, Harkins M, Kelly F, et al. Pretreatment with albuterol versus montelukast for exercise-induced bronchospasm in children. Pharmacotherapy 2008;28: 287–94.

55. Chauhan BF, Ducharme FM. Anti-leukotriene agents compared to inhaled corticosteroids in the management of recurrent and/or chronic asthma in adults and children. Cochrane Database Syst Rev 2012;(5):CD002314.

56. de Benedictis FM, Vaccher S, de Benedictis D. Montelukast sodium for exercise-induced asthma. Drugs Today (Barc) 2008;44:845–55.
57. de Benedictis FM, del Giudice MM, Forenza N, et al. Lack of tolerance to the protective effect of montelukast in exercise-induced bronchoconstriction in children. Eur Respir J 2006;28:291–5.
58. Kubavat AH, Khippal N, Tak S, et al. A randomized, comparative, multicentric clinical trial to assess the efficacy and safety of zileuton extended-release tablets with montelukast sodium tablets in patients suffering from chronic persistent asthma. Am J Ther 2013;20:154–62.
59. Lofdahl CG, Reiss TF, Leff JA, et al. Randomised, placebo controlled trial of effect of a leukotriene receptor antagonist, montelukast, on tapering inhaled corticosteroids in asthmatic patients. BMJ 1999;319:87–90.
60. Leff JA, Busse WW, Pearlman D, et al. Montelukast, a leukotriene-receptor antagonist, for the treatment of mild asthma and exercise-induced bronchoconstriction. N Engl J Med 1998;339:147–52.
61. Philip G, Swern AS, Smugar SS, et al. Baseline predictors of placebo response in exercise-induced bronchoconstriction (EIB): pooled regression analysis >from three studies of montelukast in EIB. J Asthma 2010;47:935–41.
62. Pearlman DS, van Adelsberg J, Philip G, et al. Onset and duration of protection against exercise-induced bronchoconstriction by a single oral dose of montelukast. Ann Allergy Asthma Immunol 2006;97:98–104.
63. Philip G, Nayak AS, Berger WE, et al. The effect of montelukast on rhinitis symptoms in patients with asthma and seasonal allergic rhinitis. Curr Med Res Opin 2004;20:1549–58.
64. Anderson SD, Daviskas E. The mechanism of exercise-induced asthma is.... J Allergy Clin Immunol 2000;106:453–9.
65. Anderson SD. Exercise-induced bronchoconstriction in the 21st century. J Am Osteopath Assoc 2011;111:S3–10.
66. Spooner CH, Saunders LD, Rowe BH. Nedocromil sodium for preventing exercise-induced bronchoconstriction. Cochrane Database Syst Rev 2002;(1):CD001183.
67. Spooner CH, Spooner GR, Rowe BH. Mast-cell stabilising agents to prevent exercise-induced bronchoconstriction. Cochrane Database Syst Rev 2003;(4):CD002307.
68. Kelly HW. Comparison of inhaled corticosteroids: an update. Ann Pharmacother 2009;43:519–27.
69. Tecklenburg-Lund S, Mickleborough TD, Turner LA, et al. Randomized controlled trial of fish oil and montelukast and their combination on airway inflammation and hyperpnea-induced bronchoconstriction. PLoS One 2010; 5:e13487.
70. Mickleborough TD, Lindley MR, Ionescu AA, et al. Protective effect of fish oil supplementation on exercise-induced bronchoconstriction in asthma. Chest 2006; 129:39–49.
71. Mickleborough TD, Murray RL, Ionescu AA, et al. Fish oil supplementation reduces severity of exercise-induced bronchoconstriction in elite athletes. Am J Respir Crit Care Med 2003;168:1181–9.
72. Helenius I, Lumme A, Haahtela T. Asthma, airway inflammation and treatment in elite athletes. Sports Med 2005;35:565–74.
73. Sadeh J, Israel E. Airway narrowing in athletes: a different kettle of fish? Am J Respir Crit Care Med 2003;168:1146–7.
74. Cohen HA, Neuman I, Nahum H. Blocking effect of vitamin C in exercise-induced asthma. Arch Pediatr Adolesc Med 1997;151:367–70.

75. Tecklenburg SL, Mickleborough TD, Fly AD, et al. Ascorbic acid supplementation attenuates exercise-induced bronchoconstriction in patients with asthma. Respir Med 2007;101:1770–8.
76. Schachter EN, Schlesinger A. The attenuation of exercise-induced bronchospasm by ascorbic acid. Ann Allergy 1982;49:146–51.
77. Chinellato I, Piazza M, Sandri M, et al. Serum vitamin D levels and exercise-induced bronchoconstriction in children with asthma. Eur Respir J 2011;37: 1366–70.
78. Stickland MK, Rowe BH, Spooner CH, et al. Effect of warm-up exercise on exercise-induced bronchoconstriction. Med Sci Sports Exerc 2011;44(3):383–91.
79. Millqvist E, Bake B, Bengtsson U, et al. Prevention of asthma induced by cold air by cellulose-fabric face mask. Allergy 1995;50:221–4.
80. Millqvist E, Bengtsson U, Lowhagen O. Combining a beta2-agonist with a face mask to prevent exercise-induced bronchoconstriction. Allergy 2000;55:672–5.
81. Karakatsani A, Analitis A, Perifanou D, et al. Particulate matter air pollution and respiratory symptoms in individuals having either asthma or chronic obstructive pulmonary disease: a European multicentre panel study. Environ Health 2012; 11:75. http://dx.doi.org/10.1186/1476-069X-11-75.

Assessment of EIB
What You Need to Know to Optimize Test Results

Sandra D. Anderson, PhD, DSc, MD(Hon)[a],*, Pascale Kippelen, PhD[b]

KEYWORDS

- Exercise hyperpnea • Dry air • Voluntary hyperpnea • Mannitol
- Bronchial provocation

KEY POINTS

- Respiratory symptoms are poor predictors of either the presence or the severity of exercise-induced bronchoconstriction (EIB).
- There are many factors affecting the response to exercise, such as workload, ventilation, humidity, temperature, and time since medication.
- There is a high rate of negative test results using exercise ergometers in a laboratory setting.
- Surrogates for exercise have been developed to identify the potential for EIB in the laboratory setting.
- Eucapnic voluntary hyperpnea is a very potent and sensitive test to identify EIB and is recommended to identify EIB in elite athletes or in regular exercisers with suspected mild EIB.
- Challenge with mannitol dry powder aerosol, which uses prepacked capsules of increasing doses, reduces the risk of large decreases in the forced expiratory volume in the first second of expiration, helps to identify the presence of currently active asthma, and detects the potential for EIB.

BACKGROUND TO THE NEED TO IDENTIFY EXERCISE-INDUCED BRONCHOCONSTRICTION

"Exercise-induced asthma and exercise-induced bronchoconstriction (EIB) are the terms used to describe the transient increase in airways resistance that follows vigorous exercise."[1] EIB occurs most commonly in people with clinically recognized asthma. History and symptoms cannot be relied on to predict EIB either in adults (**Fig. 1**)[2] or children.[3] In one study, 40% of children considered well controlled by a

---

Funding Sources: Nil.
Conflict of Interest: Yes (S.D. Anderson); Nil (P. Kippelen).
[a] Department of Respiratory and Sleep Medicine, Royal Prince Alfred Hospital, Camperdown, New South Wales 2050, Missenden road, Australia; [b] Centre for Sports Medicine & Human Performance, Brunel University, Kingston Lane, Uxbridge, Middlesex UB8 3PH, UK
* Corresponding author.
E-mail address: sandra.anderson@sydney.edu.au

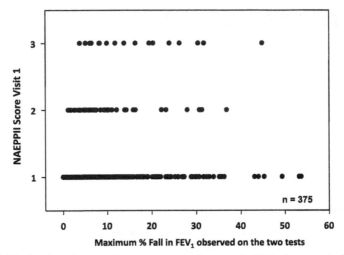

Fig. 1. Individual values for the highest percent decrease in FEV₁ documented after 2 exercise tests in relation to the National Asthma Education and Prevention Program (NAEP-PII) asthma severity score at visit 1. Score 1 = symptoms 2 or less times per week; score 2 = symptoms 2 or more times a week but less than 1 time a day; score 3 = symptoms daily. (*From* Anderson SD, Pearlman DS, Rundell KW, et al. Reproducibility of the airway response to an exercise protocol standardized for intensity, duration, and inspired air conditions, in subjects with symptoms suggestive of asthma. Respir Res 2010;11:120; with permission.)

questionnaire had EIB[4]; in another study, 40% of children with EIB had never had a diagnosis of asthma.[5] EIB also occurs in people without other symptoms of asthma, particularly elite athletes.[2,6,7] In elite athletes, self-reported symptoms related to exercise are neither sensitive nor specific for identifying EIB (**Table 1**).[2,8–11] An overdiagnosis and underdiagnosis of EIB from symptoms was realized when investigators started to measure the airway response to exercise in athletes with and without symptoms. The move away from symptoms to lung function measurement to diagnose EIB was facilitated by sporting bodies requesting objective evidence of asthma or EIB to justify the use of a beta₂ agonist aerosol before a sporting event.[12] Further, the recent large surveys on exercise-related symptoms reported in both adults[13] and children[14] in the United States suggest that objective measurement is required to identify EIB so that appropriate treatment can be prescribed.[15]

Table 1
The sensitivity, specificity, PPV, and NPV for respiratory symptoms to predict EIB

	Sensitivity %	Specificity %	PPV %	NPV %
Cough	61	65	38	83
Wheeze	17	82	25	74
Chest tightness	20	80	26	74
Excess mucus	22	85	33	76

EIB is defined as a decrease in the FEV₁ of 10% or more following actual or simulated competition exercise in elite athletes.
Based on the findings of Rundell et al.[2]
Abbreviations: NPV, negative predictive value; PPV, positive predictive value.

WHAT WE NEED TO KNOW TO IDENTIFY EIB

To develop successful protocols and reduce the possibility of false-negative tests, it is necessary to understand the stimulus and mechanism whereby exercise narrows the airways in susceptible people. This understanding also explains why surrogates for exercise, such as eucapnic voluntary hyperpnea (EVH) and inhaled mannitol, have been used successfully to identify the potential for EIB.

The stimulus for EIB is water loss, by evaporation, from the airway surface in humidifying large volumes of air in a short time (**Fig. 2**). This water loss cools the larger airways (>2 mm) and may increase the osmolarity of the airway surface liquid because of its small volume (<1 mL).[16] Inspiring cool dry air enhances the possibility of EIB, and inspiring warm humid air reduces the possibility and may even prevent EIB.[17] Exercise of high intensity is needed[18] to identify EIB because it determines ventilation; the higher the ventilation, the greater the rate of water loss. The duration of exercise is also important. It cannot be too long because of the high intensity of exercise or too short because it will not result in sufficient water loss. In combination with the intensity of exercise and inspired air conditions, duration determines the number of generations of airways required to heat and to humidify the inspired air. The greater the number of generations, the greater the surface area of the airways involved in the exercise response. Exercising under conditions that require recruiting the small airways[19] to heat and to humidify the air increases the chances of identifying EIB. The small airways have a high density of the mast cells[20] and are an important source of mediators of bronchoconstriction.

The mechanism whereby the airways narrow is thought to relate to both the osmotic and thermal effects of evaporative water loss.[21] Although water can rapidly return to the airway surface, a transient increase in osmolarity of the airway surface liquid will occur if the rate of water loss exceeds the rate of return.[19] This transient hyperosmolar environment favors the release of mediators from cells near the airway surface.[22,23] These mediators include prostaglandins (PGs), leukotrienes (LTs), and histamine, which can cause the bronchial smooth muscle to relax (PGE_2) during the first few

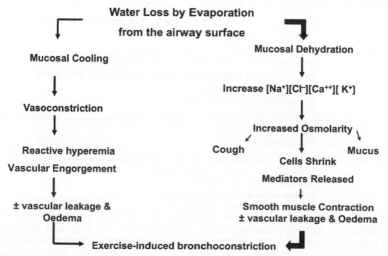

Fig. 2. The stimulus to exercise-induced bronchoconstriction is the water loss by evaporation from the airways surface in conditioning large volumes of air in a short time. The mechanism for airway narrowing relates to the thermal (cooling) and osmotic effects of this water loss.

minutes of exercise in all patients and then to contract (PGD_2, LTs, and histamine) in those with EIB.[21,24] For this reason, medications that inhibit the production or release of these mediators or antagonize their effect need to be withheld for the appropriate time **(Table 2)**. Further, patients should not have exercised within 2 hours[25] and preferably 4 hours of a test because a state of refractoriness during that period occurs in 50% of patients with EIB.[26] Even warm-up exercise can induce refractoriness.[27]

During exercise under temperate or cold conditions, the airways cool because of the latent heat of vaporization in humidifying the inspired air. The colder the inspired air is during exercise, the greater the possibility for the thermal effects to enhance the severity of EIB. The thermal effects involve a reactive hyperemia of the bronchial vasculature, which is an event that follows the vasoconstriction in response to airway cooling.[28] This reactive hyperemia may also be accompanied by increased vascular permeability and mucosal edema. As previously discussed,[29] these events may not only serve to cause narrowing in their own right but may also amplify the effects of airway narrowing arising from bronchial smooth muscle contraction. The interplay of the thermal and osmotic effects is important in the assessment of cold-weather athletes who may need to exercise under conditions that reproduce their symptoms.[30]

To optimize the chance of identifying EIB in untrained patients in a laboratory requires measuring the forced expiratory volume in the first second of expiration (FEV_1) before and at frequent intervals after exercising. The exercise should preferably

Table 2	
Medications and their required withholding times before challenge by exercise, EVH, or mannitol to reduce the possibility of a false-negative test result and optimize the possibility of finding a positive test result	
Time to Withhold	**Medication**
8 h	Short-acting β_2 agonists (eg, *albuterol, salbutamol, levalbuterol terbutaline*) Inhaled nonsteroidal antiinflammatory agents Cromones (eg, *sodium cromoglycate, nedocromil sodium*)
12 h	Inhaled corticosteroids (eg, *beclomethasone dipropionate, budesonide, fluticasone propionate, ciclesonide*) Ipratropium bromide
24 h	Inhaled corticosteroids plus long-acting β_2 agonists (eg, *fluticasone and salmeterol, budesonide and formoterol*) Long-acting β_2 agonists (eg, *salmeterol, eformoterol*) Theophylline
72 h	Tiotropium bromide Antihistamines (eg, *cetirizine, fexofenadine, and loratadine*)
4 d	Leukotriene-receptor antagonists (eg, *montelukast sodium*) Nonsteroidal antiinflammatory (eg, *indomethacin, ibuprofen*)

Foods: Ingestion of caffeine-containing foods, such as coffee, tea, cola, and chocolate, may decrease bronchial hyperresponsiveness. These substances should be withheld on the day of the test.

Other factors that may confound results: Smoking and vigorous exercise should not be undertaken on the day of the test.

Abbreviations: HR, heart rate; HRmax, predicted maximum heart rate; VE, ventilation.

involve running (rather than cycling) and should last for 6 to 8 minutes. Patients should breathe dry air via the mouth with the nose clipped and exercise intensely enough to achieve a minute ventilation more than 21 times the baseline FEV_1 (in liters) by 4 minutes, but preferably within the first 2 minutes, and maintain this level until the end of exercise. In the absence of a measure of ventilation, heart rate can be used. The target heart rate should be between 85% and 95% of the predicted maximum for the duration of the test and preferably more than 95% predicted for the last 4 minutes.[18] Protocols that have met these requirements for both running and cycling have been used successfully in laboratories or in the field.[5,10,18,30–32]

There is a high frequency of negative exercise results in those tested in a laboratory for suspected EIB.[31,33,34] This high frequency has resulted in fewer exercise tests being performed these days. Screening tests, in the field, for EIB have also had a low yield in some studies.[35] In part, this may be explained by the inadequacy of the exercise task, variable inspired air conditions, or the lack of attention to the conditions preceding the test, particularly recent exercise or the withholding of medication (see **Table 2**; **Table 3**).

Elite athletes are a special case in that sport-specific exercise in the field, under the appropriate conditions, may be required in the event of negative results of exercise tests or surrogates for exercise in the laboratory.[2,6,10] The thermal and vascular effects are expected to be the greatest under conditions of inspiring air of subfreezing temperatures (such as in winter sports), less important when breathing warm humid air (such as during swimming),[36,37] and absent under conditions of breathing hot dry air.[38,39]

HOW IS THE DIAGNOSIS OF EIB MADE?

A diagnosis of EIB is commonly made on the measurement of an abnormal reduction in the FEV_1 after exercise. The FEV_1 does not need to be accompanied by a full forced vital capacity maneuver. Measurements of the FEV_1 are usually made in duplicate or triplicate 5, 10, 15, 20, and 30 minutes after exercise, with the best FEV_1 value at each

Table 3 Key determinants of the airway response to exercise challenge	
Factors that Enhance the Possibility of EIB	Factors that Reduce the Possibility of EIB
Inspiring cold dry air	Inspiring warm humid air
Exercise of high intensity (VE >21*FEV₁ or HR >85%–95% pred HRmax within 2–4 min)	Exercise of low intensity (VE <22 × FEV₁ or HR <85% pred HRmax)
Duration of 6–8 min	Duration of less than 6 min or more than 8 min
Constant load exercise with rapid (in the first 2 min) workload increment	Incremental exercise protocol
Recent exposure to allergens	Strenuous exercise within 2–4 h before testing
Recent exposure to irritants or high densities of particulate matters	Warm-up exercise
Recent URTI or chest infection	Ingestion of caffeine-containing foods (eg, coffee, tea, cola, and chocolate) on the day of testing
	Inappropriate withholding time of drugs (cf **Table 2**)
	Out-of-season testing (for athletes only)

Abbreviations: HR, heart rate; HRmax, predicted maximum heart rate; URTI, upper respiratory tract infection; VE, ventilation.

time point being recorded. Earlier and more frequent measurements may be required to identify and avoid severe bronchoconstriction. The lowest value for the FEV_1 is usually observed within 15 minutes after exercise and recovers spontaneously within 30 to 60 minutes. Inhalation of a $beta_2$ agonist bronchodilator is recommended if there is a need to enhance recovery to the baseline FEV_1. A decrease in the FEV_1 after exercise of 10% or more from the pre-exercise value "is generally accepted as abnormal," but a cutoff of 15% or more is often used when exercise has been performed in the field.[40] The severity of EIB is expressed as the maximum percent decrease in the FEV_1 after exercise, and suggested grades of severity are given in **Table 4**. For elite athletes to identify EIB, a decrease of 10% or more in the FEV_1 is preferable at 2 consecutive time points (eg, 5 and 10 minutes after exercise). This practice reduces the possibility of a false-positive result from recording a low FEV_1 immediately at the end of exercise because of respiratory muscle fatigue.[41]

A decrease in the FEV_1 of 10% and 15% from the baseline is close to the 95% confidence interval observed in healthy subjects in the laboratory[42,43] and the field.[5,44] A value of 13% has been reported to provide the optimal sensitivity (63%) and specificity (94%) for identifying children with asthma and young adults.[45] The choice of cutoff will be determined by the investigator's need to be either more sensitive or more specific. Although a 10% decrease in the FEV_1 is acceptable for sporting bodies seeking clearance to use an inhaled $beta_2$ agonist, a value of 20% has been suggested to be included in a clinical trial to assess new drugs for EIB.[46]

VARIABILITY IN THE RESPONSE TO EXERCISE

Since the early studies in EIB 50 years ago, variability of the airway response to exercise has been recognized.[47] There is a recent report in 373 subjects with signs and symptoms of asthma but without a definite diagnosis who performed running exercises on 2 occasions within 2 to 4 days under the optimal conditions described earlier.[32] In 19% of the subjects, a decrease in the FEV_1 of 10% or more was documented after both tests. The mean of the highest percent decrease in the FEV_1 was 24.7% ± 9.7%, leaving the diagnosis of EIB in no doubt. For 24% of the subjects, only one test was positive, with the mean highest decrease being 14.3% ± 4.8%. For 57% of the subjects, the 2 tests were 10% or less with the mean of the highest percent decrease being 4.9% ± 2.9%. A value of 0% was assumed in 55 of the 210 subjects who had only an increase in the FEV_1 in response to exercise. The 5-times difference in the mean percent decrease in those with 2 positive tests and those with 2 negative tests suggests that 2 concordant test results may be useful to include or exclude a definitive diagnosis of EIB.

The variability in the percent decrease in the FEV_1 on the 2 test days was ± 9.7% in the 278 adults, ± 13.4% in the 95 children, and ± 14.6% for the 72 subjects with 2 positive exercise tests (with an FEV_1 decrease of 10% or more) (**Fig. 3**). This variability

Table 4 Classification of severity of EIB	
Degree of Severity of EIB	**Maximum Percent Decrease in FEV_1 After Exercise**
Mild	≥10% but <25%
Moderate	≥25% but <50%
Severe	≥50% for steroid-naïve patients ≥30% for steroid-treated patients

A suggested classification for severity of EIB based on the percent decrease in FEV_1.

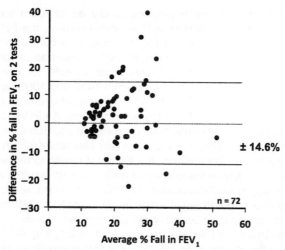

Fig. 3. Reproducibility of the percent decrease in FEV_1 measured after 8 minutes of running exercise of high intensity while breathing dry air by mouth. The difference between values for the percent decrease in FEV_1 on the 2 exercise tests performed within 2.6 ± 3.2 days in relation to the average value on the 2 tests for those 72 subjects who had a 10% or more decrease following both exercise tests. The interval defines the 95% probability that the difference between a single measurement and the true value for the subject is within that range. (*From* Anderson SD, Pearlman DS, Rundell KW, et al. Reproducibility of the airway response to an exercise protocol standardized for intensity, duration, and inspired air conditions, in subjects with symptoms suggestive of asthma. Respir Res 2010;11:120; with permission.)

in the percent decrease in the FEV_1 needs to be considered when selecting a subject for inclusion in a drug trial.

Seasonal differences can contribute to the variability of EIB.[48,49] Although variability in the percent decrease is recognized when conditions of the inspired air alone are altered, it may also be important if the environmental conditions are altered.[50] Thus, exercising in subfreezing conditions may enhance responses via a facial reflex.[51,52] These subfreezing conditions, although uncommon, have been used in a laboratory environment.[30,53] Other factors that can affect the exercise outcome are recent exposure to allergens or irritants or to high densities of particulate matter.[54–56]

During exercise testing, other conditions than EIB may cause a turbulent sound in the tracheal area. Inspiratory stridor,[57] vocal cord dysfunction,[58] or laryngeal obstruction[59] have all been reported to masquerade as EIB. It is important to consider these as a cause of symptoms (especially wheeze) if an exercise or surrogate challenge proves negative and there is no significant bronchodilator response to inhaling a beta$_2$ agonist.[60]

SURROGATE TESTS TO IDENTIFY POTENTIAL FOR EIB
EVH

The many factors that determine the outcome of an exercise test and the inherent variability of EIB prompted the development of surrogates that could be more easily standardized for use in a hospital or office laboratory. That exercise itself was not necessary to elicit an airway response to hyperpnea with dry air was recognized in the 1970s. One test protocol, standardized for evaluating defense force recruits and involving 6 minutes of voluntary hyperpnea of dry air at room temperature, has become the most widely used (**Table 5**).[61] As with exercise, the FEV_1 is measured and the maximum percent decrease in the FEV_1 usually occurs within 10 minutes of finishing the test. A value of 10% or more has been taken as abnormal, based on the finding of a specificity of 90% and a sensitivity of 63% for identifying patients with asthma. A decrease in the FEV_1 of more than 14% was 100% specific for identifying patients with asthma.[62] The variability for the percent decrease to EVH between 2 tests is reported within $\pm 6\%$.[63] The fixed concentration of 4.9% to 5.0% carbon dioxide (CO_2) allows eucapnia at ventilations between 40 and 105 L/min.[64]

This EVH test has been increasingly used to test elite athletes[65] in addition to defense force recruits.[66] For elite athletes, the EVH test needs to be performed during the training season to enhance the chance of a positive test result,[67] and a sustained 10% or more decrease in the FEV_1 is used as criteria for a positive test.[68] For athletes and recruits, 6 minutes of breathing at a high level of ventilation (30 times the FEV_1) is used as a target to reduce the possibility of false-negative results. Because this high ventilation can lead to a severe percent decrease in the FEV_1 (**Fig. 4**),[69] it is recommended for use only in those who exercise regularly and intensely at high ventilation.[70] Because of the high potency of the test, EVH is often used to exclude EIB in elite athletes, especially in those with suspected upper respiratory tract dysfunction or dysfunctional breathing.

For those who do not exercise regularly, the potency of the stimulus using EVH can be reduced by decreasing the target ventilation to 17 to 21 times the FEV_1. Provided the ventilation is 21 or more times the baseline FEV_1 (in liters) for 6 to 8 minutes, it should be a valid test to exclude EIB in most untrained patients whose ventilation during exercise is unlikely to exceed this level.[31] Using a standard 6-minute protocol, 81% of 178 patients achieved a diagnostic test.[71] Women were less likely to achieve the target ventilation of 21 times the FEV_1 compared with men. For many untrained women, however, a ventilation of 17.5 or more times the FEV_1 would be the maximum level achieved during exercise.[31]

There are many advantages in using EVH to identify EIB in the laboratory, particularly for athletes. Providing the resistance of the equipment is low and permits high flow, voluntary hyperpnea of dry air is less stressful than exercise-induced hyperpnea, particularly at high ventilation. The duration of the ventilation and the temperature of the air inspired can be varied if required to evaluate the conditions under which exercise is performed (eg, cold air and so forth). Importantly, the target ventilation is based on the FEV_1 of the individual patient and is not dependent on muscle power of the limbs. Although it is easy to set up a circuit to perform an EVH test, attention should

Table 5 Protocol for EVH for identifying EIB	
Measurement	FEV_1 before and 5, 10, and 15 min after EVH and as required
Target ventilation	30 times[a] or 21 times[b] FEV_1
Duration	6 min
Inspired air	Dry air containing 4.9% to 5.0% CO_2, 21% O_2, and balance N_2 inhaled at room temperature
Positive response	FEV_1 percent decrease 10% or more preferably at 2 consecutive time points

[a] For those who exercise intensely, Anderson et al, 2001.[70]
[b] For untrained subjects, Brummel et al, 2009.[71]

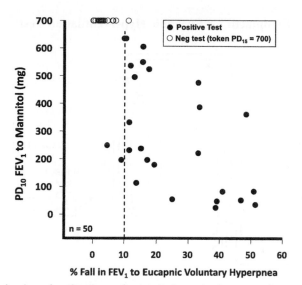

Fig. 4. Individual values for the dose of mannitol required to provoke a 10% decrease in FEV$_1$ (PD$_{10}$) in relation to the maximum percent decrease in FEV$_1$ after 6 minutes EVH of dry air at room temperature in elite athletes. (*Modified from* Holzer K, Anderson SD, Chan HK, et al. Mannitol as a challenge test to identify exercise-induced bronchoconstriction in elite athletes. Am J Respir Crit Care Med 2003;167:534–47; with permission.)

be given to minimize the dead space and to ensure a low resistance in the circuit (**Fig. 5**).[70] To overcome the limitation in ventilation set by the use of preprepared gas mixtures, a commercial system can be used that mixes the gases and monitors the fraction of CO$_2$ in inspired air and ventilation (up to 220 L/min) during challenge (EucapSys SMTEC, Switzerland).

EVH is more sensitive to detect the potential for EIB compared with exercise[6,72] and mannitol when using the same cutoff point of 10%.[69] The higher sensitivity for EVH to identify EIB likely relates to the very rapid increase (within seconds) in the rate of ventilation to the target value compared with exercise whereby minutes are required. For some patients, the dry air is an irritant to the throat and causes them to cough, so water should be provided. As with exercise, the EVH test is associated with an increase in the urinary concentration of PGs and LTs.[73,74] Care should be taken to withhold medications and abide by the same pretesting conditions as exercise (see **Tables 2** and **3**).

In one study, in all but a few athletes responsive to EVH, the PC$_{20}$ to methacholine was 2 μmol or less.[63] However, there is probably no role for methacholine challenge to identify EIB. The reason relates to the high frequency of methacholine responsiveness in those without EIB[10,75] and a low frequency of methacholine responsiveness in some groups with positive responses to EVH.[8,66] The high frequency of methacholine hyperresponsiveness in elite athletes has been attributed to airway injury.[76,77] A low frequency of methacholine hyperresponsiveness was recently reported by the US Army whereby the EVH test was positive in 26 patients negative to a methacholine challenge,[66] confirming earlier studies whereby athletes were EVH positive and methacholine negative.[8,78] In these groups, the FEV$_1$ is frequently close to or more than 100% predicted. This value may be relevant because the prevalence of hyperresponsiveness to methacholine decreases as the FEV$_1$ percent predicted increases.[79] Importantly, the mediators associated with hyperpnea and hyperosmolar challenges, namely, the PGs and LTs, are 100 and 1000 times as potent as methacholine in

Equipment for Eucapnic Hyperventilation Test

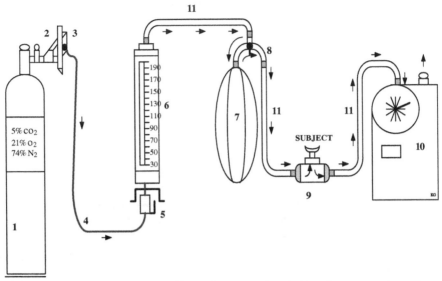

Fig. 5. Some equipment used to perform the eucapnic voluntary hyperpnea test. The gas cylinder contains 4.9-5% carbon dioxide, 21% oxygen, balance nitrogen (1). A regulator (2) a demand resuscitator 30-150 L/min (3) with high pressure tubing (4) and a demand valve in the fully open position, (5) allows the required flow of gas, to meet the target ventilation, to pass through a rotameter (6) via a three way tap (8) that allows gas to simultaneously enter and leave the large meteorological balloon (7) that acts as a reservoir. The subject inhales the dry gas via wide bore tubing (11) and a large low resistance low dead space two way valve (9) as close to the target ventilation as possible and exhales through a meter (10) that measures ventilation. (*From* Anderson SD, Argyros GJ, Magnussen H, et al. Provocation by eucapnic voluntary hyperpnoea to identify exercise induced bronchoconstriction. Br J Sports Med 2001;35:344–7; with permission.)

causing bronchoconstriction.[80] Therefore, small concentrations of PGs and LTs released during exercise or EVH may provoke a 10% or more decrease in the FEV_1 in some patients negative to methacholine.

Hyperosmolar Aerosols

Hyperosmolar saline was developed as a bronchial provocation test during the 1980s. When it was observed that patients with asthma with EIB could have an attack of asthma provoked by inhaling hyperosmolar aerosols,[81] the tests were standardized and became used as surrogates for exercise.[82,83] However, there were limitations in that a large-volume ultrasonic nebulizer was needed, and the dose of the aerosol delivered could differ widely between patients and over time, depending on the inspiratory flow through the nebulizer and the age of the piezoelectric crystal.[84] The technical and hygienic limitations associated with the correct use of the 4.5% saline test were overcome by the development of a dry powder of mannitol for inhalation.

Mannitol as a dry powder was chosen as the osmotic stimulus because it is stable at high relative humidity, has many medical applications, and was generally regarded as a safe molecule.[85] Mannitol caused the release of mast cell histamine in vitro, and this release was enhanced in the presence of anti–immunoglobulin E.[86] Mannitol inhalation in vivo has been shown to be associated with the same increase in urinary concentration of PGs and LTs as those observed in response to exercise or EVH.[73,74,87,88]

The mannitol test kit (known as Aridol or Osmohale; Pharmaxis Inc, Exton, PA) contains prepacked capsules with increasing doses and an inhaler device, so there is no preparation or cleanup time required (**Table 6**). The dose response protocol reduces the risk of large decreases in the FEV_1 that can occur unexpectedly following exercise and EVH. A positive test is a 15% decrease in the FEV_1 at a cumulative dose of 635 mg or a 10% decrease between doses. The test result is expressed as the provoking dose to induce a 15% decrease in the FEV_1 (PD_{15}) and is a measure of sensitivity. This value is based on the 95% confidence interval documented in healthy subjects.[89] The repeatability of the PD_{15} is within ± 1 doubling dose both in adults and children.[90,91] The response dose ratio (RDR), a measure of reactivity, is calculated taking the final percent decrease in the FEV_1 after challenge divided by the cumulative dose of mannitol to provoke that percent decrease in the FEV_1. The 95% confidence interval for RDR in healthy subjects is a 0.004% decrease in the FEV_1 per milligram.[89] A 0% decrease after mannitol is taken as 0.1% in calculating the RDR.[89]

Most patients will cough during the mannitol challenge, but in 71% this is occasional; in 13% it causes a delay in administering the capsule, and in 1.3% the challenge cannot be completed.[89] The mannitol test has regulatory approval and is available in 26 countries, including the United States, Europe, Australia, and South Korea, to identify bronchial hyperresponsiveness. As with hyperosmolar saline, sputum can be induced with mannitol inhalation and collected for analysis.[92]

In groups of well-defined patients, hyperresponsiveness to mannitol has been shown to have high specificity for a clinical diagnosis of asthma (95%), with a sensitivity of approximately 60%.[89,93,94] This sensitivity increases to 89% when the use of inhaled corticosteroids (ICS) is taken into account.[89] This finding means that like exercise, a positive mannitol test is consistent with the diagnosis of asthma, but a negative test does not exclude asthma. Most studies comparing responses to exercise and mannitol show concordant test results both for children at 84%[95] and 80%[96] and for adults at 74%.[34] Mannitol had a sensitivity of 59% and 69% to identify a 10% or 15% decrease in the FEV_1 in a group of patients with symptoms but without a definite diagnosis of asthma when 2 identical exercise tests were performed within a few days.[34] However, the frequency of a positive mannitol response was 1.41 times that of a 10% or more decrease on the first exercise test and 1.65 times greater than a 15% decrease.[34,97]

Table 6
Mannitol provocation test kit[a] protocol

Inhaled agent	Dry powder mannitol
Increasing doses	0, 5, 10, 20, 40, 80, 160, 160, 160 mg
Measurements	FEV_1 before and 1 min after dose with highest value for FEV_1 recorded
Positive response	Decrease FEV_1 15% or more or 10% between doses
Expression of result	
Sensitivity	PD_{15}
Reactivity	Response dose ratio
Recovery	Bronchodilator or spontaneous

The time of testing should be kept to a minimum to progressively increase the osmotic gradient and less than 35 minutes.
[a] Commercially available as Aridol or Osmohale.

There are individuals in whom a mannitol test is positive and EIB or EVH test is negative and vice versa.[34,69] For those individuals with a positive mannitol test, the diagnosis is confirmed and the potential to get EIB is identified. The study in subjects with exercise wheeze is a good example of this, whereby 36 of 39 (92%) subjects tested positive to mannitol but only 14 (36%) had EIB to the exercise protocol.[98] When the exercise or EVH test is positive at a 10% or more decrease in the FEV_1 and the mannitol test is negative, the different cutoff points should be kept in mind and the percent decreases in the FEV_1 compared. Further, if exercise or EVH tests are performed with cold air inspirate, borderline airway responses may be entirely mediated by reactive hyperemia, with ensuing vascular engorgement and edema in the mucosa and submucosa (but without inflammatory mediator release).[28] Some investigators have reported a 10% decrease or PD_{10} to mannitol to compare responses with EVH (see **Fig. 4**),[69,99] whereas others have compared mannitol and exercise in children using a 15% decrease for both tests.[95,96] In addition, it is useful to calculate the reactivity to mannitol (ie, RDR) and relate it to the maximum percent decrease after exercise, which is also an index of reactivity.

A positive response to mannitol is consistent with other indices of inflammation and was observed in 82% of those with eosinophilic asthma.[100] The response to mannitol was greater in those with a higher exhaled nitric oxide.[101] In 252 patients with asthma treated with ICS, the frequency of a positive mannitol test was 51%,[102] a value similar to that reported for exercise.[31] As with a negative exercise test, caution is needed when interpreting a negative mannitol test in those being treated with ICS. In these patients, the negative test is likely caused by a reduction in inflammatory cell number[103] or concentration of mediators rather than a loss of sensitivity of the bronchial smooth muscle, which remains hyperresponsive to methacholine even after months of treatment with high doses of ICS.[104]

In elite athletes, one might commonly encounter a positive methacholine test result but a negative result to challenge with mannitol, exercise, or EVH. A possible reason for this is that epithelial injury can result in a positive methacholine test because the access of the methacholine to the smooth muscle is enhanced by the injury. The same athlete may have no significant airway inflammation and, as a result, have negative tests to mannitol, exercise, or EVH.[10] For this reason, it is not appropriate to make a diagnosis of asthma or identify the potential for EIB in elite athletes from a positive methacholine test result alone.

REFERENCES

1. Freed AN, Anderson SD. Exercise-induced bronchoconstriction. Human models. In: Kay AB, editor. Allergy & allergic diseases. Oxford (United Kingdom): Blackwell Scientific Publications; 2008. p. 806–20.
2. Rundell KW, Im J, Mayers LB, et al. Self-reported symptoms and exercise-induced asthma in the elite athlete. Med Sci Sports Exerc 2001;33:208–13.
3. De Baets F, Bodart E, Dramaix-Wilmet M, et al. Exercise-induced respiratory symptoms are poor predictors of bronchoconstriction. Pediatr Pulmonol 2005; 39:301–5.
4. Madhuban AA, Driessen JM, Brusse-Keizer MG, et al. Association of the asthma control questionnaire with exercise-induced bronchoconstriction. J Asthma 2011;3:275–8.
5. Haby MM, Peat JK, Mellis CM, et al. An exercise challenge for epidemiological studies of childhood asthma: validity and repeatability. Eur Respir J 1995;8: 729–36.

6. Mannix ET, Manfredi F, Farber MO. A comparison of two challenge tests for identifying exercise-induced bronchospasm in figure skaters. Chest 1999;115:649–53.
7. Parsons JP, Kaeding C, Phillips G, et al. Prevalence of exercise-induced bronchospasm in a cohort of varsity college athletes. Med Sci Sports Exerc 2007; 39:1487–92.
8. Holzer K, Anderson SD, Douglass J. Exercise in elite summer athletes: challenges for diagnosis. J Allergy Clin Immunol 2002;110:374–80.
9. Dickinson JW, Whyte GP, McConnell AK, et al. Mid expiratory flow versus FEV1 measurements in the diagnosis of exercise-induced asthma in elite athletes. Thorax 2006;61:111–4.
10. Sue-Chu M, Brannan JD, Anderson SD, et al. Airway hyperresponsiveness to methacholine, adenosine5-monophosphate, mannitol, eucapnic voluntary hyperpnoea and field exercise challenge in elite cross country skiers. Br J Sports Med 2010;44:827–32.
11. Parsons JP. Exercise-induced bronchospasm: symptoms are not enough. Expert Rev Clin Immunol 2009;5:357–9.
12. Anderson SD, Fitch K, Perry CP, et al. Responses to bronchial challenge submitted for approval to use inhaled beta2 agonists prior to an event at the 2002 Winter Olympics. J Allergy Clin Immunol 2003;111:44–9.
13. Parsons JP, Craig TJ, Stoloff SW, et al. Impact of exercise-related respiratory symptoms in adults with asthma: Exercise-Induced Bronchospasm Landmark National Survey. Allergy Asthma Proc 2011;32:431–7.
14. Ostrom NK, Eid NS, Craig TJ, et al. Exercise-induced bronchospasm in children with asthma in the United States: results from the Exercise-Induced Bronchospasm Landmark Survey. Allergy Asthma Proc 2011;32:425–30.
15. Weiler JM, Anderson SD, Randolph C, et al. Pathogenesis, prevalence, diagnosis, and management of exercise-induced bronchoconstriction: a practice parameter. Ann Allergy Asthma Immunol 2010;105:S1–46.
16. Anderson SD, Daviskas E, Smith CM. Exercise-induced asthma: a difference in opinion regarding the stimulus. Allergy Proc 1989;10:215–26.
17. Anderson SD, Schoeffel RE, Follet R, et al. Sensitivity to heat and water loss at rest and during exercise in asthmatic patients. Eur J Respir Dis 1982;63:459–71.
18. Carlsen KH, Engh G, Mørk M. Exercise induced bronchoconstriction depends on exercise load. Respir Med 2000;94:750–5.
19. Daviskas E, Gonda I, Anderson SD. Local airway heat and water vapour losses. Respir Physiol 1991;84:115–32.
20. Carroll ML, Carroll NG, Gundersen HJ, et al. Mast cell densities in bronchial biopsies and small airways are related. J Clin Pathol 2011;64:394–8.
21. Anderson SD, Daviskas E. The mechanism of exercise-induced asthma is…. J Allergy Clin Immunol 2000;106:453–9.
22. Hjoberg J, Folkerts G, van Gessel SB, et al. Hyperosmolarity-induced relaxation and prostaglandin release in guinea pig trachea in vitro. Eur J Pharmacol 2000; 398:303–7.
23. Gulliksson M, Palmberg L, Nilsson G, et al. Release of prostaglandin D2 and leukotriene C4 in response to hyperosmolar stimulation of mast cells. Allergy 2006;61:1473–9.
24. Anderson SD, Kippelen P. Exercise-induced bronchoconstriction: pathogenesis. Curr Allergy Asthma Rep 2005;5:116–22.
25. Edmunds A, Tooley M, Godfrey S. The refractory period after exercise-induced asthma: its duration and relation to the severity of exercise. Am Rev Respir Dis 1978;117:247–54.

26. Schoeffel RE, Anderson SD, Gillam I, et al. Multiple exercise and histamine challenge in asthmatic patients. Thorax 1980;35:164–70.

27. Reiff DB, Choudry NB, Pride NB, et al. The effect of prolonged submaximal warm-up exercise on exercise-induced asthma. Am Rev Respir Dis 1989;139:479–84.

28. McFadden ER, Lenner KA, Strohl KP. Postexertional airway rewarming and thermally induced asthma. J Clin Invest 1986;78:18–25.

29. Anderson SD, Holzer K. Exercise-induced asthma: is it the right diagnosis in elite athletes? J Allergy Clin Immunol 2000;106:419–28.

30. Stensrud T, Berntsen S, Carlsen KH. Exercise capacity and exercise-induced bronchoconstriction (EIB) in a cold environment. Respir Med 2007;101:1529–36.

31. Anderson SD, Lambert S, Brannan JD, et al. Laboratory protocol for exercise asthma to evaluate salbutamol given by two devices. Med Sci Sports Exerc 2001;33:893–900.

32. Anderson SD, Pearlman DS, Rundell KW, et al. Reproducibility of the airway response to an exercise protocol standardized for intensity, duration, and inspired air conditions, in subjects with symptoms suggestive of asthma. Respir Res 2010;11:120.

33. Rundell KW, Wilber RL, Szmedra L, et al. Exercise-induced asthma screening of elite athletes: field vs laboratory exercise challenge. Med Sci Sports Exerc 2000;32:309–16.

34. Anderson SD, Charlton B, Weiler JM, et al. Comparison of mannitol and methacholine to predict exercise-induced bronchoconstriction and a clinical diagnosis of asthma. Respir Res 2009;10:4.

35. Hallstrand TS, Curtis JR, Koepsell TD, et al. Effectiveness of screening examinations to detect unrecognised exercise-induced bronchoconstriction. J Pediatr 2002;141:343–9.

36. Clearie KL, Williamson PA, Vaidyanathan S, et al. Disconnect between standardized field-based testing and mannitol challenge in Scottish elite swimmers. Clin Exp Allergy 2010;40:731–7.

37. Romberg K, Bjermer L, Tufvesson E. Exercise but not mannitol increases Clara cell protein (CC16) in elite swimmers. Respir Med 2011;105:31–6.

38. Aitken ML, Marini JJ. Effect of heat delivery and extraction on airway conductance in normal and in asthmatic subjects. Am Rev Respir Dis 1985;131:357–61.

39. Anderson SD, Schoeffel RE, Black JL, et al. Airway cooling as the stimulus to exercise-induced asthma - a re-evaluation. Eur J Respir Dis 1985;67:20–30.

40. Crapo RO, Casaburi R, Coates AL, et al. Guidelines for methacholine and exercise challenge testing - 1999. Am J Respir Crit Care Med 2000;161:309–29.

41. Johnson BD, Babcock MA, Suman OE, et al. Exercise-induced diaphragmatic fatigue in healthy humans. J Physiol 1993;460:385–405.

42. Kattan M, Thomas CM, Keens TG, et al. The response to exercise in normal and asthmatic children. J Pediatr 1978;92:718–21.

43. Custovic A, Arifhodzic N, Robinson A, et al. Exercise testing revisited. The response to exercise in normal and atopic children. Chest 1994;105:1127–32.

44. Backer V, Dirksen A, Bach-Mortensen N, et al. The distribution of bronchial responsiveness to histamine and exercise in 527 children and adolescents. J Allergy Clin Immunol 1991;88:68–76.

45. Godfrey S, Springer C, Bar-Yishay E, et al. Cut-off points defining normal and asthmatic bronchial reactivity to exercise and inhalation challenges in children and young adults. Eur Respir J 1999;14:659–68.

46. Food and Drug Administration Guidance for Industry. Available at: http://www. fda.gov./cder/guidance. Accessed October 27, 2012.

47. Anderson S, Seale JP, Ferris L, et al. An evaluation of pharmacotherapy for exercise-induced asthma. J Allergy Clin Immunol 1979;64:612–24.

48. Helenius IJ, Tikkanen HO, Haahtela T. Occurrence of exercise induced broncho-spasm in elite runners: dependence on atopy and exposure to cold air and pollen. Br J Sports Med 1998;32:125–9.

49. Choi IS, Ki WJ, Kim TO, et al. Seasonal factors influencing exercise-induced asthma. Allergy Asthma Immunol Res 2012;4:192–6.

50. Koskela H, Tukiainen H, Kononoff A, et al. Effect of whole-body exposure to cold and wind on lung function in asthmatic patients. Chest 1994;105:1728–31.

51. Koskela H, Tukiainen H. Facial cooling, but not nasal breathing of cold air, in-duces bronchoconstriction: a study in asthmatic and healthy subjects. Eur Respir J 1995;8:2088–93.

52. Zeitoun M, Wilk B, Matsuzaka A, et al. Facial cooling enhances exercise-induced bronchoconstriction in asthmatic children. Med Sci Sports Exerc 2004;36:767–71.

53. Evans TM, Rundell KW, Beck KC, et al. Cold air inhalation does not affect the severity of EIB after exercise or eucapnic voluntary hyperventilation. Med Sci Sports Exerc 2005;37:544–9.

54. Henriksen JM. Exercise-induced bronchoconstriction. Seasonal variation in children with asthma and in those with rhinitis. Allergy 1986;41:468–70.

55. Karjalainen J, Lindqvist A, Laitenen LA. Seasonal variability of exercise-induced asthma especially out-doors. Effect of birch pollen allergy. Clin Exp Allergy 1989;19:273–9.

56. Rundell KW, Spiering BA, Baumann JM, et al. Bronchoconstriction provoked by exercise in a high-particulate-matter environment is attenuated by montelukast. Inhal Toxicol 2005;17:99–105.

57. Rundell KW, Spiering BA. Inspiratory stridor in elite athletes. Chest 2003;123:468–74.

58. McFadden ER, Zawadski DK. Vocal cord dysfunction masquerading as exercise-induced asthma. A physiologic cause for "choking" during athletic activities. Am J Respir Crit Care Med 1996;153:942–7.

59. Christensen PM, Thomsen SF, Rasmussen N, et al. Exercise-induced laryngeal obstructions: prevalence and symptoms in the general public. Eur Arch Otorhi-nolaryngol 2011;268:1313–9.

60. Abu-Hasan M, Tannous B, Weinberger M. Exercise-induced dyspnea in children and adolescents: if not asthma then what? Ann Allergy Asthma Immunol 2005; 94:366–71.

61. Argyros GJ, Roach JM, Hurwitz KM, et al. Eucapnic voluntary hyperventilation as a bronchoprovocation technique. Development of a standardized dosing schedule in asthmatics. Chest 1996;109:1520–4.

62. Hurwitz KM, Argyros GJ, Roach JM, et al. Interpretation of eucapnic voluntary hyperventilation in the diagnosis of asthma. Chest 1995;108:1240–5.

63. Stadelmann K, Stensrud T, Carlsen KH. Respiratory symptoms and bronchial responsiveness in competitive swimmers. Med Sci Sports Exerc 2011;43:375–81.

64. Phillips YY, Jaeger JJ, Laube BL, et al. Eucapnic voluntary hyperventilation of compressed gas mixture. A simple system for bronchial challenge by respiratory heat loss. Am Rev Respir Dis 1985;131:31–5.

65. Fitch KD, Sue-Chu M, Anderson SD, et al. Asthma and the elite athlete: summary of the International Olympic Committee's Consensus Conference, Lausanne, Switzerland, January 22–24, 2008. J Allergy Clin Immunol 2008;122:254–60.

66. Holley AB, Cohee B, Walter RJ, et al. Eucapnic voluntary hyperpnea is superior to methacholine challenge testing for detecting airway hyperreactivity in nonathletes. J Asthma 2012;49(6):614–9.

67. Bougault V, Turmel J, Boulet LP. Airway hyperresponsiveness in elite swimmers: is it a transient phenomenon? J Allergy Clin Immunol 2011;127:892–8.

68. Bougault V, Boulet LP, Turmel J. Bronchial challenges and respiratory symptoms in elite swimmers and winter sport athletes. Chest 2010;138:31S–7S.

69. Holzer K, Anderson SD, Chan HK, et al. Mannitol as a challenge test to identify exercise-induced bronchoconstriction in elite athletes. Am J Respir Crit Care Med 2003;167:534–47.

70. Anderson SD, Argyros GJ, Magnussen H, et al. Provocation by eucapnic voluntary hyperpnoea to identify exercise induced bronchoconstriction. Br J Sports Med 2001;35:344–7.

71. Brummel NE, Mastronarde JG, Rittinger D, et al. The clinical utility of eucapnic voluntary hyperventilation testing for the diagnosis of exercise-induced bronchospasm. J Asthma 2009;46:683–6.

72. Rundell KW, Anderson SD, Spiering BA, et al. Field exercise vs laboratory eucapnic voluntary hyperventilation to identify airway hyperresponsiveness in elite cold weather athletes. Chest 2004;125:909–15.

73. Kippelen P, Larsson J, Anderson SD, et al. Effect of sodium cromoglycate on mast cell mediators during hyperpnea in athletes. Med Sci Sports Exerc 2010;42:1853–60.

74. Kippelen P, Larsson J, Anderson SD, et al. Acute effects of beclomethasone on hyperpnea-induced bronchoconstriction. Med Sci Sports Exerc 2010;42: 273–80.

75. Stensrud T, Mykland KV, Gabrielsen K, et al. Bronchial hyperresponsiveness in skiers: field test versus methacholine provocation? Med Sci Sports Exerc 2007; 39:1681–6.

76. Anderson SD, Kippelen P. Airway injury as a mechanism for exercise-induced bronchoconstriction in elite athletes. J Allergy Clin Immunol 2008;122:225–35.

77. Bougault V, Turmel J, St-Laurent J, et al. Asthma, airway inflammation and epithelial damage in swimmers and cold-air athletes. Eur Respir J 2009;33: 734–9.

78. Pedersen L, Winther S, Backer V, et al. Airway responses to eucapnic hyperpnea, exercise and methacholine in elite swimmers. Med Sci Sports Exerc 2008;40:1567–72.

79. Norval J, Perry CP, Anderson SD. Responses to methacholine and eucapnic voluntary hyperpnea in relation to baseline lung function [abstract]. Respirology 2007;12:A1.

80. O'Byrne PM. Leukotrienes in the pathogenesis of asthma. Chest 1997;111: 27S–34S.

81. Smith CM, Anderson SD. Hyperosmolarity as the stimulus to asthma induced by hyperventilation? J Allergy Clin Immunol 1986;77:729–36.

82. Smith CM, Anderson SD. Inhalation provocation tests using non-isotonic aerosols. J Allergy Clin Immunol 1989;84:781–90.

83. Riedler J, Reade T, Dalton M, et al. Hypertonic saline challenge in an epidemiological survey of asthma in children. Am J Respir Crit Care Med 1994;150: 1632–9.

84. Anderson SD, Brannan JD. Methods for 'indirect' challenge tests including exercise, eucapnic voluntary hyperpnea and hypertonic aerosols. Clin Rev Allergy Immunol 2003;24:63–90.

85. Anderson SD, Brannan J, Spring J, et al. A new method for bronchial-provocation testing in asthmatic subjects using a dry powder of mannitol. Am J Respir Crit Care Med 1997;156:758–65.
86. Eggleston PA, Kagey-Sobotka A, Schleimer RP, et al. Interaction between hyperosmolar and IgE-mediated histamine release from basophils and mast cells. Am Rev Respir Dis 1984;130:86–91.
87. Brannan JD, Gulliksson M, Anderson SD, et al. Evidence of mast cell activation and leukotriene release after mannitol inhalation. Eur Respir J 2003;22:491–6.
88. Brannan JD, Gulliksson M, Anderson SD, et al. Inhibition of mast cell PGD2 release protects against mannitol-induced airway narrowing. Eur Respir J 2006;27:944–50.
89. Brannan JD, Anderson SD, Perry CP, et al. The safety and efficacy of inhaled dry powder mannitol as a bronchial provocation test for airway hyperresponsiveness: a phase 3 comparison study with hypertonic (4.5%) saline. Respir Res 2005;6:144.
90. Brannan JD, Anderson SD, Gomes K, et al. Fexofenadine decreases sensitivity to and montelukast improves recovery from inhaled mannitol. Am J Respir Crit Care Med 2001;163:1420–5.
91. Barben J, Roberts M, Chew N, et al. Repeatability of bronchial responsiveness to mannitol dry powder in children with asthma. Pediatr Pulmonol 2003;36:490–4.
92. Wood LG, Powell H, Gibson PG. Mannitol challenge for assessment of airway responsiveness, airway inflammation and inflammatory phenotype in asthma. Clin Exp Allergy 2010;40:232–41.
93. Sverrild A, Porsbjerg C, Thomsen SF, et al. Diagnostic properties of inhaled mannitol in the diagnosis of asthma: a population study. J Allergy Clin Immunol 2009;124:928–932.e1.
94. Sverrild A, Porsbjerg C, Thomsen SF, et al. Airway hyperresponsiveness to mannitol and methacholine and exhaled nitric oxide: a random-sample population study. J Allergy Clin Immunol 2010;126:952–8.
95. Barben J, Kuehni C, Strippoli M-P, et al. Mannitol dry powder challenge in comparison with exercise-testing in children. Pediatr Pulmonol 2011;46:842–8.
96. Kersten ET, Driessen JM, van der Berg JD, et al. Mannitol and exercise challenge tests in asthmatic children. Pediatr Pulmonol 2009;44:655–61.
97. Anderson SD, Brannan JD. Bronchial provocation testing: the future. Curr Opin Allergy Clin Immunol 2011;11:46–52.
98. Cowan SC, Hewitt RS, Cowan JO, et al. Exercise-induced wheeze: fraction of exhaled nitric oxide directed management. Respirology 2010;15:683–90.
99. Aronsson D, Tufvesson E, Bjermer L. Comparison of central and peripheral airway involvement before and during methacholine, mannitol and eucapnic hyperventilation challenges in mild asthmatics. Clin Respir J 2011;5:10–8.
100. Porsbjerg C, Lund TK, Pedersen L, et al. Inflammatory subtypes in asthma are related to airway hyperresponsiveness to mannitol and exhaled NO. J Asthma 2009;46:606–12.
101. Anderson WJ, Lipworth BJ. Relationship of mannitol challenge to methacholine challenge and inflammatory markers in persistent asthmatics receiving inhaled corticosteroids. Lung 2012;90(5):513–21.
102. Brannan JD, Perry CP, Anderson SD. Mannitol test results in asthmatic adults receiving inhaled corticosteroids. J Allergy Clin Immunol 2012. [Epub ahead of print].

103. James A, Gyllfors P, Henriksson E, et al. Corticosteroid treatment selectively decreases mast cells in the smooth muscle and epithelium of asthmatic bronchi. Allergy 2012;67:958–61.
104. Reddel HK, Jenkins CR, Marks GB, et al. Optimal asthma control, starting with high doses of inhaled budesonide. Eur Respir J 2000;16:226–35.

Assessment of Exercise-Induced Bronchoconstriction in Adolescents and Young Children

Janneke C. van Leeuwen, MD[a,c],*,
Jean M.M. Driessen, MD, PhD[a,b], Elin T.G. Kersten, MD[a,c],
Bernard J. Thio, MD, PhD[a]

KEYWORDS

- Exercise-induced bronchoconstriction • Children • Adolescents
- Pulmonary function • Asthma • Exercise challenge test • Bronchial provocation test

KEY POINTS

- Adults and children show differences in exercise-induced bronchoconstriction (EIB).
- The time course of EIB is age-dependent; the younger the child, the shorter the time to maximal bronchoconstriction and the quicker the recovery from EIB.
- Many children with EIB have breakthrough EIB (bronchoconstriction starting during exercise).
- EIB symptoms are poorly recognized by children, parents, and clinicians.
- An age-adjusted exercise challenge test is the first choice test to assess EIB in children, and is feasible in children as young as 3 years.
- Alternative bronchial provocation tests are available when exercise tests cannot be performed.

INTRODUCTION

Exercise-induced bronchoconstriction (EIB) is defined as a transient narrowing of the airways that follows vigorous exercise.[1] EIB is a common manifestation of asthma in children and adolescents, occurring in up to 90% of the asthmatic children.[2,3] Its prevalence in the general pediatric population is between 6% and 20%.[2,4,5]

EIB compromises the participation of children in play and sports, and may result in a negative influence on quality of life, cardiovascular condition, and psychomotor development.[6–8]

Conflict of Interest: All authors have no conflicts of interest to disclose.
[a] Department of Pediatrics, Medisch Spectrum Twente, VKC poli 17, Haaksbergerstraat 55, Enschede 7513 ER, The Netherlands; [b] Department of Sports Medicine, Tjongerschans Hospital, Thialfweg 44, Heerenveen 8441 PW, The Netherlands; [c] Department of Pediatric Pulmonology, GRIAC Research Institute, University Medical Center Groningen, Beatrix Children's Hospital, Hanzeplein 1, Groningen 9713 GZ, The Netherlands
* Corresponding author.
E-mail address: vanleeuwen.janneke@gmail.com

In children, EIB is highly specific for asthma,[9] and because EIB reflects airway inflammation, it indicates uncontrolled asthma.[9–11] Thus the assessment of EIB in children is used to not only diagnose EIB but also monitor asthma.

TIME COURSE OF EIB IN CHILDREN

EIB is characterized as a reduction in postexercise pulmonary function.[3,12] The course of EIB in children generally consists of an initial bronchodilation early during exercise.[12] The bronchoconstriction typically begins after cessation of exercise,[4,13] but may start during exercise ("breakthrough" EIB),[14,15] and peaks 2 to 15 minutes after exercise (Fig. 1),[2,13,15,16] followed by spontaneous recovery of pulmonary function, which can last about 30 to 60 minutes.[2,13] About 50% of the children with EIB subsequently experience a refractory period, which can last between 45 minutes and 3 hours.[2,17]

Several studies showed that the course of EIB changes with age.[13,18] Vilozni and colleagues[13] systematically assessed the relationship between age and time to maximal bronchoconstriction (Nadir − t) after exercise. These investigators retrospectively reviewed data of exercise challenge tests in 4- to 18-year-old children and adolescents, and found a significant relation between age and Nadir − t ($R^2 = 0.54$, $P<.001$). The mean Nadir − t was at 5.1 ± 2.6 minutes, and none of the children reached Nadir − t later than 12 minutes after exercise.[13] Another study investigated the spontaneous recovery of pulmonary function after maximal

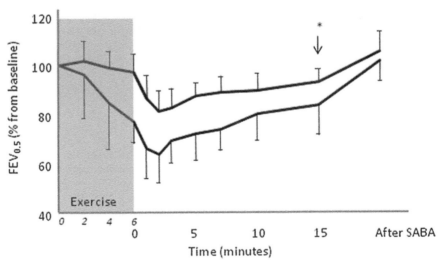

Fig. 1. Mean expiratory volume in 0.5 second ($FEV_{0.5}$) $\pm$ standard deviation during and after exercise in 5- to 7-year-old children with breakthrough exercise-induced bronchoconstriction (EIB) (ie, $\geq 13\%$ decrease in $FEV_{0.5}$ during exercise, sustained after exercise; *lower graph*) and nonbreakthrough EIB (ie, $\geq 13\%$ decrease in $FEV_{0.5}$ after exercise; *upper graph*). Note that the children with breakthrough EIB have a more severe decrease in pulmonary function and slower recovery from EIB compared with nonbreakthrough EIB, indicating severe EIB.[15] As percentage of baseline (*asterisk*) administration of 100 μg salbutamol. SABA, short-acting β-agonist (ie, salbutamol). (*Data from* van Leeuwen JC, Driessen JM, de Jongh FH, et al. Measuring breakthrough exercise induced bronchoconstriction in young asthmatic children using a jumping castle. J Allergy Clin Immunol 2012. http://dx.doi.org/10.1016/j.jaci.2012.10.014. pii:S0091-6749(12)01658-2.)

bronchoconstriction, induced by exercise and histamine, in 7- to 12-year-old children with EIB. The recovery rate (ie, % increase in forced expiratory volume in 1 second [FEV_1] per minute) for EIB decreased significantly with increasing age, in contrast to the recovery rate for histamine.[18] Thus, the younger the child, the shorter the time to maximal bronchoconstriction after exercise and the quicker the recovery from EIB.[13,18]

BREAKTHROUGH EIB IN CHILDREN

EIB has been described as airway narrowing occurring after the cessation of exercise. However, several studies assessing pulmonary function in asthmatic children during exercise have found that EIB often occurs during, and is sustained after, exercise; this is known as breakthrough EIB.[14,15,19] Breakthrough EIB (defined as a 15% decrease in FEV_1 during exercise) has been described in 8- to 15-year-old asthmatic children, occurring 6 to 10 minutes after the start of exercise and before cessation of exercise.[14] Another study, measuring $FEV_{0.5}$ during and after exercise in 5- to 7-year-old asthmatic children, showed that breakthrough EIB (defined as a 13% decrease in $FEV_{0.5}$) in this age group can even occur within 2 minutes of starting exercise, suggesting a shift of the breakthrough phenomenon with age.[15] The relation between age and time to breakthrough EIB as derived from the data from studies of van Leeuwen and colleagues[15] is shown in **Fig. 2**. Breakthrough EIB is accompanied by a more severe decrease in pulmonary function and slower recovery from EIB compared with non-breakthrough EIB, indicating severe EIB. Therefore in children, symptoms of dyspnea within minutes of starting exercise may well be caused by EIB and may result in the child quickly dropping out of play and sports.

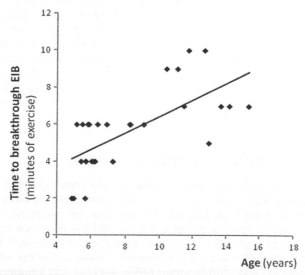

Fig. 2. Relation between age and time to breakthrough EIB, defined as a >13% decrease in FEV_1 or $FEV_{0.5}$ during exercise (N = 27). r = 0.73, P<.01. (*Data from* van Leeuwen JC, Driessen JM, de Jongh FH, et al. Monitoring pulmonary function during exercise in children with asthma. Arch Dis Child 2011;96:664–8; and van Leeuwen JC, Driessen JM, de Jongh FH, et al. Measuring breakthrough exercise induced bronchoconstriction in young asthmatic children using a jumping castle. J Allergy Clin Immunol 2012. http://dx.doi.org/10.1016/j.jaci.2012.10.014. pii:S0091-6749(12)01658-2.)

PATHOPHYSIOLOGY OF EIB IN CHILDREN

EIB is thought to be largely caused by dehydration of the respiratory mucosa during exercise-induced hyperpnea. This airway dehydration leads to hyperosmolarity of the mucosa and subsequent release of inflammatory mediators, causing bronchoconstriction.[1] Another proposed mechanism for EIB is the thermal hypothesis, which states that exercise-induced hyperpnea causes airway cooling. After exercise, when hyperpnea ceases, the airways rapidly rewarm, leading to engorgement of the hyperplastic vascular bed in the asthmatic airway wall and subsequent bronchoconstriction.[20] The quick onset of bronchoconstriction during exercise (breakthrough EIB) and the rapid recovery from EIB after exercise, as observed in young children, are not compatible with the thermal hypothesis. Indeed, rapid rewarming of the airways was not shown to enhance EIB in children.[21] The thermal phenomenon, however, may contribute to EIB and explain the protracted recovery seen in asthmatic adults, particularly those exercising in a cold environment.

Several mechanisms could explain the quick onset of EIB in young children in comparison with older children and adults. Exercise-induced hyperpnea is associated with the increased urinary excretion of inflammatory mediators.[22,23] EIB in children has been successfully inhibited by leukotriene antagonists,[24] loratadine (an antihistamine),[25] and mast-cell stabilizers, such as sodium cromoglycate and nedocromil sodium,[26] supporting a role for inflammatory mediators in EIB. Perhaps their release occurs faster in children than in adults, owing to swift changes in osmolarity. Young children may be prone to rapid airway dehydration, as their minute ventilation is relatively high and their capacity to humidify the inspired air low in comparison with adults.[27,28] Mast cells respond rapidly to a change in osmolarity, as shown many years ago.[29,30] Furthermore, the airway smooth muscle in young airways could have a shortened response and relaxation time in comparison with adolescents or adults.[16,31] This rapid hyperresponsiveness of young airways may account for breakthrough EIB and the rapid pattern of bronchoconstriction after exercise in young children.[13] Finally, breakthrough EIB could be explained by a failure of the exercise-induced release of bronchoprotective prostaglandins, such as prostaglandin E_2 as suggested by Larsson and colleagues,[32] to counterbalance the mast-cell mediators causing bronchoconstriction during exercise. Further research is necessary to clarify these mechanisms, and particularly to measure the release of bronchoconstrictive and bronchoprotective mediators in children with breakthrough and nonbreakthrough EIB.

ASSESSING EIB IN CHILDREN; RECOGNITION OF SYMPTOMS

The characteristic presenting symptoms of EIB include chest tightness, wheeze, and cough.[33,34] However, EIB in children can also be accompanied by subtle, nonspecific symptoms, such as fatigue, abdominal or chest pain, or headache.[34] It has been shown that reported symptoms do not correlate with the presence of EIB.[15,34] For example, most children with EIB cough but, as with adult athletes,[35] this symptom is not specific for EIB.[15,36] Panditi and Silverman[37] investigated the relationship between parent-reported and child-reported EIB symptoms and laboratory-diagnosed EIB, and concluded that reported symptoms weakly relate to objective measures of severity of EIB. Children seem to have a poor perception of EIB symptoms, and may fail to notice symptoms until taking part in organized sports.[16] About 50% of children with asthma who reported a negative history of EIB had a positive response to an exercise challenge test (ECT).[2] Parents' perception of the extent and severity of their children's EIB did not relate to any measurement of lung function.[37] Even clinician-observed symptoms seem to be poor predictors of EIB,[15,33] leading to both false-positive and false-negative diagnosis and treatment of EIB.

ASSESSING EIB IN CHILDREN; QUESTIONNAIRES

Asthma control questionnaires, such as the Asthma Control Questionnaire (ACQ)[38] or the (Childhood) Asthma Control Test ([C]-ACT),[39,40] are widely used and validated measures for the evaluation and control of asthma.[11,38–40] As EIB is considered to be a sign of uncontrolled asthma, one could expect a significant relationship between questionnaires and EIB.[9–11] However, the ACT failed to detect EIB in a significant percentage of 6- to 17-year-old asthmatic children.[41] A similar study investigated EIB in 5- to 7-year-old children, and showed a poor association between the C-ACT and EIB, even during provocative exercise challenges in cold, dry air.[15] Chinellato and colleagues[42] observed that nocturnal symptoms related better with EIB than symptoms, indicating activity limitations, and reinforcing the notion that the occurrence of EIB can be considered a sign of poor asthma control.[9–11] A limitation of the ACT is the lack of an exercise-specific question. The ACQ does have a distinct question regarding exercise limitations, but also showed no relation with the occurrence of EIB.[43] This study described a positive predictive value of 51% and a negative predictive value of 59% to predict EIB in adolescents, when using the ACQ cutoff points set by Juniper and colleagues.[38,43] The relationship between the individual ACQ score and exercise-induced decrease in FEV_1, as investigated by Madhuban and colleagues,[43] is shown in **Fig. 3**.

One may conclude that although EIB is one of the hallmarks of asthma in children and is a clear sign of uncontrolled asthma, children, parents, and clinicians seem to be unable to grasp its presence without testing.

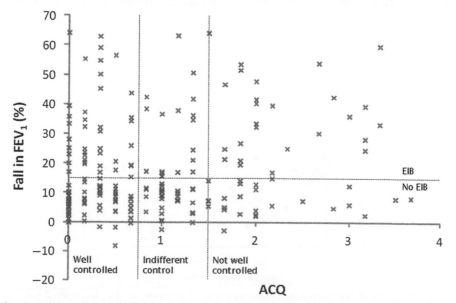

Fig. 3. Relation between asthma control questionnaire (ACQ) score and exercise-induced decrease in FEV_1, as percentage decrease from baseline (N = 200). Dotted lines represent cutoff value for EIB (ie, 15% decrease in FEV_1) and cutoff values for asthma control (<0.75 well-controlled asthma, >1.50 not well-controlled asthma). (*Data from* Madhuban AA, Driessen JM, Brusse-Keizer MG, et al. Association of the Asthma Control Questionnaire with exercise-induced bronchoconstriction. J Asthma 2011;48:275–8.)

ASSESSING EIB IN CHILDREN; EXERCISE CHALLENGE TEST

ECTs have been studied extensively and are well standardized for children older than 8 years.[5,16,44] Children younger than 8 years can perform ECTs as well, using an age-adjusted approach.[15,16,45] Vilzoni and colleagues[16] performed ECTs in children as young as 3 years.

An ECT consists of pulmonary function measurements before and after exercise. Although an ECT remains the first-choice bronchial provocation test (BPT) to assess EIB in children,[2] it should be interpreted carefully. The advantage of an ECT in the assessment of EIB is that it is a "real-life" test, providing direct insight, for both parents and clinicians, into the severity and course of a child's EIB. Especially for children, an ECT can be more enjoyable than other BPTs.

The limitation of the ECT lies in standardizing the many factors that can affect the airway response to exercise, such as the temperature and water content of the inspired air, and the duration and intensity of exercise. Insufficient attention to these important determinants of EIB may produce false-negative outcomes.[46] The airway response to exercise is moderately reproducible; the variability in the percentage decrease in FEV_1 for children is 13.4% (**Fig. 4**).[47] Therefore, more than 1 ECT may be required to include or exclude EIB.[47] This variation in airway response could be due to different factors, such as changes in intensity of exercise, environmental or dietary factors, or the intrinsic reproducibility of an ECT itself.[47] Moreover, particularly in children, variability in airway response could be the result of refracto-riness,[17,44] as children have multiple bouts of physical exercise during the day. Finally, an ECT in its current form does not have a dose response, and ECTs can trigger severe decreases in pulmonary function. To identify breakthrough EIB, the latter could be overcome when measuring pulmonary function during exercise.[14]

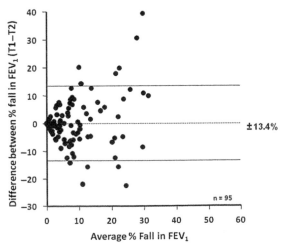

Fig. 4. Variability in the percentage exercise induced decrease in FEV_1 between 2 exercise challenge tests within 4 days in children with mild symptoms of asthma (N = 95). The interval defines the 95% probability that the difference between a single measurement and the true value for the subject is within that range. (*Reproduced from* Anderson SD, Pearlman DS, Rundell KW, et al. Reproducibility of the airway response to an exercise protocol standardized for intensity, duration, and inspired air conditions, in subjects with symptoms suggestive of asthma. Respir Res 2010;11:120; with permission.)

Exercise Challenge Test; Pulmonary Function Measurements

The most widely used guidelines for testing are from the 1999 American Thoracic Society statement, and recommend FEV_1 as the primary outcome variable for detecting EIB.[44] A postexercise decrease in FEV_1 of 10% is generally accepted as diagnostic for EIB,[44] although other cutoffs have been suggested for use in children, such as 13%[48] and 15%.[5] Alternative spirometric measures such as $FEV_{0.5}$ can be used as well,[49] as most young children are unable to perform the required full forced expiration during a total second.[15,16,49,50] In a recent study, 69% of 5- to 7-year-old children showed a baseline Tiffeneau index (FEV_1/forced vital capacity) of 90% or greater,[15] demonstrating that FEV_1 almost equaled forced vital capacity, which could reduce the usefulness of FEV_1 as an index of airway obstruction.[15,49]

The use of big-breath tests such as FEV_1 to evaluate EIB may in itself influence the obstruction, as a deep breath may lead to bronchodilatation[51] or bronchoconstriction.[52] The forced oscillation technique (FOT) does not rely on forced breathing maneuvers, and is an elegant method to analyze the patency of the airways, for example in young children unable to perform spirometry. The FOT analyzes the resistance and reactance of the airways using acoustical impedance.[53] The resistive component of respiratory impedance (Rrs) depends on the airway caliber. The reactive component of respiratory impedance (Xrs) incorporates the mass-inertive forces of the air column in the conducting airways and the elastic properties of lung periphery,[54] namely lung stiffness, intraparenchymal airway mechanics, and airway-parenchyma interdependence. The FOT has been used to evaluate EIB,[45,51,55–57] and Malmberg and colleagues[45] suggested that an increase of more than 35% in the Xrs at 5 Hz indicated the presence of EIB in young children.

Schedule of Pulmonary Function Measurements

Pulmonary function measurements should be performed before (baseline) and serially after exercise, using a standardized schedule.[44] A general recommended appropriate testing schedule is 5, 10, 15, 20, and 30 minutes after cessation of exercise.[44] However, because the time to maximal bronchoconstriction and recovery from EIB in children is age-dependent, the schedule of postexercise pulmonary function measurements should be cautiously trimmed.[13] Vilozni and colleagues[16] investigated EIB in 3- to 6-year-old children, measuring pulmonary function at 1, 2, 3, 5, 10, and 20 minutes after exercise. Maximal bronchoconstriction often occurred within 3 minutes after exercise, and could disappear as soon as 5 minutes after exercise. The investigators concluded that the exclusion of measurements up to 5 minutes after exercise may miss or underestimate the severity of the bronchoconstriction.[16] Another study measured EIB and breakthrough EIB in 5- to 7-year-old children, measuring pulmonary function at 2, 4, and 6 minutes during exercise and at 1, 2, 3, 5, 7, 10, and 15 minutes after exercise.[15] In this study the mean maximum bronchoconstriction was at 2 minutes after exercise, which corresponds to data from Vilozni and colleagues.[16] Pulmonary function in most 3- to 7-year-old children recovers within 15 to 20 minutes,[15,16] which allows earlier termination of pulmonary function measurements in comparison with an adult ECT. Moreover, young children have a short attention span and easily fatigue as a result of repeated forced breathing maneuvers. Pulmonary function measurements in this age group therefore require special attention, such as the use of incentives, comfortable position (ie, without nose clip), and skilled and patient technicians.[16,49]

Measurements of pulmonary function during exercise are feasible in children and can identify breakthrough EIB, providing a thorough assessment of EIB in children.[14,15]

Modes of Exercise

The exercise performed during an ECT should be of sufficient duration and intensity to provoke a bronchoconstriction response, and preferably be standardized.[58] Current guidelines recommend 6 to 8 minutes of exercise with 4 to 6 minutes at near-maximum target (heart rate of 80%–90% of maximum [220 minus age]).[44] The preferred mode of exercise for an ECT in schoolchildren is the treadmill or cycle ergometer.[16,44] In children younger than 8 years, free-run tests are often used to asses EIB.[16,45] However, in young children the duration of running seems to be limited by age, and forced running might be overwhelming, which could lead to a high test-failure percentage and possibly underdiagnosis of EIB.[15,16] Alternative modes of exercise in these young children could basically be any exercise that is sustainable, safe, and enjoyable, and during which heart rate can be reasonably maintained above 80% of predicted maximum.[15] For example, one study successfully performed ECTs in 5- to 7-year-old children using a jumping castle, an inflatable platform that children are familiar with and can safely jump on.[15] During exercise, climatic conditions (air temperature and humidity) should be stable. Optimally, the water content of the inspired air should be less than 10 mg/L,[44,58,59] which can be accomplished by testing in an air-conditioned room.

ASSESSING EIB IN CHILDREN; ALTERNATIVE CHALLENGES

Although an ECT is usually the first choice to diagnose EIB, alternative tests that mimic the dehydrating effect of exercise-induced hyperpnea on the airways are available.[60] Standardized BPTs are used to assess bronchial hyperresponsiveness (BHR) through the administration of bronchoconstrictor stimuli. BPTs are classified into 2 categories: (1) indirect challenges, whereby a stimulus acts on intermediate cells, such as mast cells, to induce airflow limitation through the release of pro-inflammatory mediators; and (2) direct challenges, whereby a pharmaceutical agent such as methacholine or histamine is the provoking agent that induces expiratory airflow limitation through a direct action on effector cells, such as airway smooth muscle and mucous glands.[61]

The response to a direct stimulus reflects airway smooth-muscle function and airway caliber. Although these direct tests are sensitive for identifying BHR in an asthmatic population, they are not specific for asthma. For example, methacholine challenges in girls have a sensitivity of between 71% and 77% and a specificity of 53% to 69% for detecting asthma.[62] Subjects with other pulmonary diseases and even healthy subjects may demonstrate BHR to these stimuli.[48,63] The response to an indirect stimulus is more closely associated with current airway inflammation, as it reflects the presence and active state of inflammatory cells, such as mast cells and eosinophils, in the airway.[61,64] Indirect BPTs are therefore highly specific for diagnosing asthma that is currently active, and for this reason can be used to monitor the response to anti-inflammatory treatment.[65,66] As exercise is considered an indirect stimulus, other indirect challenges, such as mannitol, eucapnic voluntary hyperpnea (EVH), hypertonic saline, and adenosine monophosphate (AMP), are preferred over direct challenges for assessing EIB.[65,67]

Mannitol

The inhalation of dry-powder mannitol was developed as an indirect BPT, as mannitol can mimic the airway drying provoked by exercise by dehydrating the airway surface and thereby triggering the release of inflammatory mediators.[68] A mannitol test is performed according to a standard protocol, with inhalation of increasing doses of mannitol.[60,67–69] The test ends when a 15% or greater decrease in FEV_1 from baseline or a 10% or greater decrease between subsequent doses occurs, or the cumulative dose of 635 mg mannitol has been administered. Sensitivity to mannitol is expressed as the provoking dose to cause a 15% decrease in FEV_1 ($PD_{15\%}$). Reactivity to mannitol is expressed as the response dose ratio, defined as the final percent decrease in FEV_1 divided by the total cumulative dose of mannitol to induce such a decrease in FEV_1. A mannitol challenge is associated with mast-cell release of mediators and an increase in urinary concentration of inflammatory mediators.[70] A mannitol challenge is a suitable alternative to an ECT.[71] With a negative predictive value of 91%, it is a useful method to exclude EIB in children.[72] A mannitol test has the built-in safety feature of a progressive dose-response challenge, so the test can be stopped before severe decreases in FEV_1 occur. A majority of patients (85.3%)[68] experience coughing during the mannitol challenge, which in some cases causes a delay in the challenge. As the rate of delivery of the osmotic stimulus is an important determinant for the severity of induced BHR, this could lead to false-negative tests.

Eucapnic Voluntary Hyperpnea

EVH mimics the airway drying provoked by exercise by voluntary hyperpnea of dry air at a high ventilation rate. A sustained 10% or greater decrease in FEV_1 following EVH is considered consistent with a diagnosis of EIB. A positive EVH test is associated with an increase in urinary excretion of the same inflammatory mediators as exercise.[22] Although EVH tests with dry air, and especially with cold air, are feasible in children as young as 2 years,[73,74] it is technically a difficult test to conduct properly in children. EVH has the potential to provoke severe bronchoconstriction and should only be performed by highly trained specialists, with safety equipment available.

Hypertonic Saline

Nebulized hypertonic saline acts by increasing airway surface liquid osmolarity, triggering sensitized cells (in particular, mast cells) to release inflammatory mediators.[60,67,69] During a hypertonic saline challenge, an aerosol of 4.5% hypertonic saline is inhaled for progressively increasing intervals of 1 to 8 minutes.[67,69] The test is terminated after a 15% or greater decrease in FEV_1 is observed, or when a total minimum dose of 23 g has been administered in 15.5 minutes.[67,69] As with any osmotic stimulus, cough occurs in the majority of patients (73.5%) with 4.5% saline.[68] Children who are positive to hypertonic saline are 4.3 times more likely to have EIB than those who are negative.[75] In 348 asthmatic children, the sensitivity of a $PD_{15\%}$ to 4.5% saline to identify EIB (defined as $\geq$10% decrease in FEV_1) was 53.9%, with a specificity of 87.6%.[75] In very young children, hypertonic saline may be easier than EVH or exercise to administer. An advantage of hypertonic saline over exercise and EVH is that it can be used to collect sputum for mediator and cellular analysis concurrently with the measurement of BHR.[67] Furthermore, the hypertonic saline challenge produces a dose-dependent response, thereby preventing a severe decrease in FEV_1. A disadvantage of the hypertonic saline challenge is that many factors can alter the output of the aerosol, such as the temperature, the volume of fluid in the nebulizer, the tidal volume of the subject, and the size of the valves and tubing.[69]

Adenosine Monophosphate

AMP challenge is a nonosmotic indirect BPT. Dry crystalline AMP powder is dissolved in 0.9% saline and is administered in progressively doubling concentrations via a nebulizer. After inhalation, AMP dephosphorylates into adenosine. Adenosine is a protein that binds to specific G-protein–coupled receptors on the cell surface of mast cells, stimulating degranulation with subsequent release of inflammatory mediators.[60,69] The response to AMP is expressed as the provoking concentration to cause a 20% decrease in FEV_1.[60,69]

AMP challenge is used in research into mechanisms rather than as a routine BPT. There are limited data available on the sensitivity and specificity of AMP challenge in identifying EIB.[76]

SUMMARY

Adults and children show marked differences in EIB; the younger the child, the shorter the time to maximal bronchoconstriction and the quicker the recovery from EIB. The weak relationship between exercise-induced symptoms and EIB as measured in ECTs in children urges the use of BPTs. An age-adjusted ECT is the first-choice test to assess EIB in children, and is feasible in children as young as 3 years. An ECT is a real-life and revealing test for both children and their parents. Assessing pulmonary function during exercise to identify breakthrough EIB can provide additional important information about the severity of a child's EIB.

REFERENCES

1. Anderson SD, Daviskas E. The mechanism of exercise-induced asthma is.... J Allergy Clin Immunol 2000;106:453–9.
2. Milgrom H, Taussig LM. Keeping children with exercise-induced asthma active. Pediatrics 1999;104:e38.
3. Cropp GJ. Grading, time course, and incidence of exercise-induced airway obstruction and hyperinflation in asthmatic children. Pediatrics 1975;56:868–79.
4. Carlsen KH, Carlsen KC. Exercise-induced asthma. Paediatr Respir Rev 2002;3: 154–60.
5. Haby MM, Peat JK, Mellis CM, et al. An exercise challenge for epidemiological studies of childhood asthma: validity and repeatability. Eur Respir J 1995;8: 729–36.
6. Merikallio VJ, Mustalahti K, Remes ST, et al. Comparison of quality of life between asthmatic and healthy school children. Pediatr Allergy Immunol 2005;16:332–40.
7. Croft D, Lloyd B. Asthma spoils sport for too many children. Practitioner 1989; 233:969–71.
8. Vahlkvist S, Inman MD, Pedersen S. Effect of asthma treatment on fitness, daily activity and body composition in children with asthma. Allergy 2010;65:1464–71.
9. Godfrey S, Springer C, Noviski N, et al. Exercise but not methacholine differentiates asthma from chronic lung disease in children. Thorax 1991;46:488–92.
10. Anderson SD. Exercise-induced asthma in children: a marker of airway inflammation. Med J Aust 2002;177(Suppl):S61–3.
11. Bateman ED, Hurd SS, Barnes PJ, et al. Global strategy for asthma management and prevention: GINA executive summary. Eur Respir J 2008;31:143–78.
12. Anderson SD, Silverman M, Konig P, et al. Exercise-induced asthma. A Review. Br J Dis Chest 1975;69:1–39.
13. Vilozni D, Szeinberg A, Barak A, et al. The relation between age and time to maximal bronchoconstriction following exercise in children. Respir Med 2009;103:1456–60.
14. van Leeuwen JC, Driessen JM, de Jongh FH, et al. Monitoring pulmonary function during exercise in children with asthma. Arch Dis Child 2011;96:664–8.
15. van Leeuwen JC, Driessen JM, de Jongh FH, et al. Measuring breakthrough exercise induced bronchoconstriction in young asthmatic children using a jumping castle. J Allergy Clin Immunol 2012. http://dx.doi.org/10.1016/j.jaci.2012.10.014. pii:S0091-6749(12)01658-2.

16. Vilozni D, Bentur L, Efrati O, et al. Exercise challenge test in 3- to 6-year-old asthmatic children. Chest 2007;132:497–503.
17. Schoeffel RE, Anderson SD, Gillam I, et al. Multiple exercise and histamine challenge in asthmatic patients. Thorax 1980;35:164–70.
18. Hofstra WB, Sterk PJ, Neijens HJ, et al. Prolonged recovery from exercise-induced asthma with increasing age in childhood. Pediatr Pulmonol 1995;20: 177–83.
19. Anderson SD, Daviskas E, Smith CM. Exercise-induced asthma: a difference in opinion regarding the stimulus. Allergy Proc 1989;10:215–26.
20. McFadden ER. Hypothesis: exercise-induced asthma as a vascular phenomenon. Lancet 1990;14(335):880–3.
21. Smith CM, Anderson SD, Walsh S, et al. An investigation of the effects of heat and water exchange in the recovery period after exercise in children with asthma. Am Rev Respir Dis 1989;140:598–605.
22. Kippelen P, Larsson J, Anderson SD, et al. Effect of sodium cromoglycate on mast cell mediators during hyperpnea in athletes. Med Sci Sports Exerc 2010; 42:1853–60.
23. Nagakura T, Obata T, Shichijo K, et al. GC/MS analysis of urinary excretion of 9α,11β-PGF2 in acute and exercise-induced asthma in children. Clin Exp Allergy 1998;28:181–6.
24. Kemp JP, Dockhorn RJ, Shapiro GG, et al. Montelukast once daily inhibits exercise-induced bronchoconstriction in 6- to 14-year-old children with asthma. J Pediatr 1998;133:424–8.
25. Baki A, Orhan F. The effect of loratadine in exercise-induced asthma. Arch Dis Child 2002;86:38–9.
26. Spooner CH, Spooner GR, Rowe BH. Mast-cell stabilising agents to prevent exercise-induced bronchoconstriction. Cochrane Database Syst Rev 2003;(4):CD002307.
27. Miller MD, Marty MA, Arcus A, et al. Differences between children and adults: implications for risk assessment at California EPA. Int J Toxicol 2002;21:403–18.
28. Tabka Z, Ben Jebria A, Vergeret J, et al. Effect of dry warm air on respiratory water loss in children with exercise-induced asthma. Chest 1988;94:81–6.
29. Eggleston PA, Kagey-Sobotka A, Schleimer RP, et al. Interaction between hyperosmolar and IgE-mediated histamine release from basophils and mast cells. Am Rev Respir Dis 1984;130:86–91.
30. Gulliksson M, Palmberg L, Nilsson G, et al. Release of prostaglandin D2 and leukotriene C4 in response to hyperosmolar stimulation of mast cells. Allergy 2006;61:1473–9.
31. Chitano P, Murphy TM. Maturational changes in airway smooth muscle shortening and relaxation. Implications for asthma. Respir Physiol Neurobiol 2003;137: 347–59.
32. Larsson J, Perry CP, Anderson SD, et al. The occurrence of refractoriness and mast cell mediator release following mannitol-induced bronchoconstriction. J Appl Physiol 2011;110:1029–35.
33. De Baets F, Bodart E, Dramaix-Wilmet M, et al. Exercise-induced respiratory symptoms are poor predictors of bronchoconstriction. Pediatr Pulmonol 2005; 39:301–5.
34. Storms WW. Review of exercise-induced asthma. Med Sci Sports Exerc 2003;35: 1464–70.
35. Rundell KW, Im J, Mayers LB, et al. Self-reported symptoms and exercise-induced asthma in the elite athlete. Med Sci Sports Exerc 2001;33:208–13.

36. Driessen JM, van der Palen J, van Aalderen WM, et al. Inspiratory airflow limitation after exercise challenge in cold air in asthmatic children. Respir Med 2012; 106:1362–8.
37. Panditi S, Silverman M. Perception of exercise induced asthma by children and their parents. Arch Dis Child 2003;88:807–11.
38. Juniper EF, Bousquet J, Abetz L, et al, GOAL Committee. Identifying 'well-controlled' and 'not well-controlled' asthma using the Asthma Control Questionnaire. Respir Med 2006;100:616–21.
39. Liu AH, Zeiger R, Sorkness C, et al. Development and cross-sectional validation of the Childhood Asthma Control Test. J Allergy Clin Immunol 2007;119:817–25.
40. Nathan RA, Sorkness CA, Kosinski M, et al. Development of the asthma control test: a survey for assessing asthma control. J Allergy Clin Immunol 2004;113: 59–65.
41. Rapino D, Consilvio NP, Scaparrotta A, et al. Relationship between exercise-induced bronchospasm (EIB) and asthma control test (ACT) in asthmatic children. J Asthma 2011;48:1081–4.
42. Chinellato I, Piazza M, Sandri M, et al. Evaluation of association between exercise-induced bronchoconstriction and childhood asthma control test questionnaire scores in children. Pediatr Pulmonol 2012;47:226–32.
43. Madhuban AA, Driessen JM, Brusse-Keizer MG, et al. Association of the Asthma Control Questionnaire with exercise-induced bronchoconstriction. J Asthma 2011;48:275–8.
44. Crapo RO, Casaburi R, Coates AL, et al. American Thoracic Society. Guidelines for methacholine and exercise challenge testing—1999. Am J Respir Crit Care Med 2000;161:309–29.
45. Malmberg LP, Makela MJ, Mattila PS, et al. Exercise-induced changes in respiratory impedance in young wheezy children and nonatopic controls. Pediatr Pulmonol 2008;43:538–44.
46. Anderson SD, Kippelen P. Assessment and prevention of exercise-induced bronchoconstriction. Br J Sports Med 2012;46:391–6.
47. Anderson SD, Pearlman DS, Rundell KW, et al. Reproducibility of the airway response to an exercise protocol standardized for intensity, duration, and inspired air conditions, in subjects with symptoms suggestive of asthma. Respir Res 2010; 11:120.
48. Godfrey S, Springer C, Bar-Yishay E, et al. Cut-off points defining normal and asthmatic bronchial reactivity to exercise and inhalation challenges in children and young adults. Eur Respir J 1999;14:659–68.
49. Arets HG, Brackel HJ, van der Ent CK. Forced expiratory manoeuvres in children: do they meet ATS and ERS criteria for spirometry? Eur Respir J 2001;18: 655–60.
50. American Thoracic Society/European Respiratory Society Working Group on Infant and Young Children Pulmonary Function Testing. An official American Thoracic Society/European Respiratory Society statement: pulmonary function testing in preschool children. Am J Respir Crit Care Med 2007;175:1304–45.
51. Schweitzer C, Vu LT, Nguyen YT, et al. Estimation of the bronchodilatory effect of deep inhalation after a free run in children. Eur Respir J 2006;28:89–95.
52. Scichilone N, Permutt S, Togias A. The lack of the bronchoprotective and not the bronchodilatory ability of deep inspiration is associated with airway hyperresponsiveness. Am J Respir Crit Care Med 2001;163:413–9.
53. Oostveen E, MacLeod D, Lorino H, et al. ERS task force on respiratory impedance measurements. The forced oscillation technique in clinical

practice: methodology, recommendations and future developments. Eur Respir J 2003;22:1026–41.

54. Smith HJ, Reinhold P, Goldman MD. Forced oscillation technique and impulse oscillometry. Eur Respir Mon 2005;31:72–105.

55. Driessen JM, Nieland H, van der Palen JA, et al. Effects of a single dose inhaled corticosteroid on the dynamics of airway obstruction after exercise. Pediatr Pulmonol 2011;46:849–56.

56. Boccaccino A, Peroni DG, Pietrobelli A, et al. Forced oscillometry is applicable to epidemiological settings to detect asthmatic children. Allergy Asthma Proc 2007; 28:170–3.

57. Wesseling GJ, Vanderhoven-Augustin IM, Wouters EF. Forced oscillation technique and spirometry in cold air provocation tests. Thorax 1993;48:254–9.

58. Godfrey S. Bronchial hyper-responsiveness in children. Paediatr Respir Rev 2000;1:148–55.

59. Anderson SD, Schoeffel RE, Follet R, et al. Sensitivity to heat and water loss at rest and during exercise in asthmatic patients. Eur J Respir Dis 1982;63:459–71.

60. Rundell KW, Slee JB. Exercise and other indirect challenges to demonstrate asthma or exercise-induced bronchoconstriction in athletes. J Allergy Clin Immunol 2008;122:238–46.

61. Joos GF, O'Connor B, Anderson SD, et al. Indirect airway challenges. Eur Respir J 2003;21:1050–68.

62. Liem JJ, Kozyrskyj AL, Cockroft DW, et al. Diagnosing asthma in children: what is the role for methacholine bronchoprovocation testing? Pediatr Pulmonol 2008;43: 481–9.

63. Carlsen KH, Engh G, Mørk M, et al. Cold air inhalation and exercise-induced bronchoconstriction in relationship to methacholine bronchial responsiveness: different patterns in asthmatic children and children with other chronic lung diseases. Respir Med 1998;92:308–15.

64. Duong M, Subbarao P, Adelroth E, et al. Sputum eosinophils and the response of exercise-induced bronchoconstriction to corticosteroid in asthma. Chest 2008; 133:404–11.

65. Cockcroft D, Davis B. Direct and indirect challenges in the clinical assessment of asthma. Ann Allergy Asthma Immunol 2009;103:363–9.

66. Brannan JD. Bronchial hyperresponsiveness in the assessment of asthma control. Chest 2010;138:11S–7S.

67. Weiler JM, Anderson SD, Randolph C, et al. Pathogenesis, prevalence, diagnosis, and management of exercise-induced bronchoconstriction: a practice parameter. Ann Allergy Asthma Immunol 2010;105:S1–47.

68. Brannan JD, Anderson SD, Perry CP, et al, Aridol Study Group. The safety and efficacy of inhaled dry powder mannitol as a bronchial provocation test for airway hyperresponsiveness: a phase 3 comparison study with hypertonic (4.5%) saline. Respir Res 2005;6:144.

69. Anderson SD, Brannan JD. Methods for 'indirect' challenge tests including exercise, eucapnic voluntary hyperpnea and hypertonic aerosols. Clin Rev Allergy Immunol 2003;24:27–54.

70. Brannan JD, Gulliksson M, Anderson SD, et al. Evidence of mast cell activation and leukotriene release after mannitol inhalation. Eur Respir J 2003;22:491–6.

71. Barben J, Kuehni C, Strippoli MP, et al. Mannitol dry powder challenge in comparison with exercise-testing in children. Pediatr Pulmonol 2011;46:842–8.

72. Kersten ET, Driessen JM, van der Berg JD, et al. Mannitol and exercise challenge tests in asthmatic children. Pediatr Pulmonol 2009;44:655–61.

73. Nielsen KG, Bisgaard H. Hyperventilation with cold versus dry air in 2- to 5-year-old children with asthma. Am J Respir Crit Care Med 2005;171:238–41.
74. Zach M, Polgar G, Kump H, et al. Cold air challenge of airway hyperreactivity in children: practical application and theoretical aspects. Pediatr Res 1984;18: 469–78.
75. Riedler J, Reade T, Dalton M, et al. Hypertonic saline challenge in an epidemiologic survey of asthma in children. Am J Respir Crit Care Med 1994;150:1632–9.
76. Avital A, Godfrey S, Springer C. Exercise, methacholine, and adenosine 5'-monophosphate challenges in children with asthma: relation to severity of the disease. Pediatr Pulmonol 2000;30:207–14.

Airways Disorders and the Swimming Pool

Valérie Bougault, PhD[a],*, Louis-Philippe Boulet, MD[b]

KEYWORDS

- Swimming • Asthma • Chlorine • Exercise • Airways

KEY POINTS

- Physical activity has beneficial effects on the health of subjects with asthma. Among different sports swimming is the less asthmogenic.
- Although controversial, some authors suggested that regular chlorinated swimming pools attendance favors the development of allergic diseases and asthma in infants, young children, adolescents, and recreational swimmers.
- Lifeguards and competitive swimmers, who are frequently exposed to a chlorine environment, are particularly concerned by an increase in occupational asthma in the former, and airway disorders, especially airway hyperresponsiveness, rhinitis, and allergies.
- Intense swimming training in a chlorinated swimming pool on a recurrent basis may promote the development of a specific phenotype of asthmatic airways.
- Simple hygienic measures could help reduce the quantity of chlorine by-products released in the swimming pool environment, and possible airway disorders in swimmers.

INTRODUCTION

Swimming is a common physical activity worldwide for recreational and competitive purposes. In western countries, swimming is often part of schools sports curricula, especially for young children. Swimming is also recommended for those having a body-weight limitation to physical activity, elderly subjects, or those with disabilities or injury. The humid and warm atmosphere encountered in indoor pools is considered particularly beneficial for patients affected by respiratory diseases, such as asthma, and swimming is associated with less exercise-induced bronchoconstriction (EIB) than other types of sport.[1,2]

Funding Sources: None.
Conflict of Interest: None.
[a] Department of Sport sciences and Physical education, Université Droit et Santé Lille 2, E.A. 4488, Lille F-59000, France; [b] Research centre, Institut Universitaire de Cardiologie et de Pneumologie, 2725 chemin Ste Foy, Québec, Québec G1V 4G5, Canada
* Corresponding author. Université du Droit et de la Santé Lille 2, FSSEP, 9 rue de l'université, Ronchin 59790, France.
E-mail address: valerie.bougault@univ-lille2.fr

Immunol Allergy Clin N Am 33 (2013) 395–408
http://dx.doi.org/10.1016/j.iac.2013.02.008
0889-8561/13/$ – see front matter © 2013 Elsevier Inc. All rights reserved.

immunology.theclinics.com

Physical activities performed in the water are predominantly performed in indoor swimming pools, partly for reasons related to the climate. Despite the high efficiency of chlorine and its derivatives to control nearly all viral and bacterial water contamination, there is controversy regarding the possible deleterious effects of chlorine disinfection on the development of asthma and allergic diseases.[3,4] Indeed, increasing evidence suggests a relationship between regular attendance at chlorinated swimming pools and the development of airway injury, allergic diseases, and asthma.[5–10] Although it is generally accepted that elite swimmers and lifeguards are the most likely to be affected by such exposure,[11–21] the possibility that young children or recreational swimmers frequently exposed to such an environment will develop airway disorders remains controversial.[3,4]

This article discusses the current benefits and risks of swimming in chlorine-disinfected swimming pools for subjects with and without asthma, and provides an overview of the current knowledge on the effects of indoor pool environments on the airways of swimmers.

BENEFITS OF SWIMMING IN SUBJECTS WITH ASTHMA OR EIB

EIB and exercise-induced asthma, which is evidenced by a fall in forced expiratory volume in 1 second (FEV_1) after exercises, can be observed in up to 90% of subjects with asthma.[22,23] However, regular physical activity improves global health of these subjects, reduces exercise-induced asthma symptoms, and should be part of asthma management.[24] In subjects with asthma, swimming is associated with a lower frequency of EIB compared with running or cycling, when exercise is performed at same the level of intensity.[1,25] For this reason, swimming is often recommended because of its lower asthmogenicity. The precise mechanism underlying this protective effect is still unclear but it is most likely related to the influence of high humidity and warm temperature of the air inhaled during exercise.[1,25] Additional mechanisms have been proposed. For example the hydrostatic pressure shifts blood volume from the legs to the chest, possibly counteracting excessive respiratory heat and water loss.[26] Through chest compression, the immersion-related pressure may also help to reduce the expiratory effort.[26] Another mechanism is the bronchodilation induced by the CO_2 retention associated with hypoventilation secondary to a controlled breathing pattern during swimming.[27]

Influence of Humid and Warm Environment on the Airways

The respiratory heat and water loss associated with high minute ventilation during exercise seems to be responsible for EIB in subjects who are hyperresponsive.[1,25,28] Although a reduction of airway temperature may influence EIB,[22] the osmotic consequences of respiratory water loss are thought to be most important.[29] The increase in airway osmolarity induces a movement of water across the airway epithelium to the airway surface, to replace the respiratory water loss. An increase in osmolarity in the local environment favors the release of inflammatory mediators, such as histamine, prostaglandins, and leukotrienes from inflammatory cells. It is these mediators that are thought to cause bronchoconstriction. Both ventilation and degree of humidification of air inhaled during exercise determine the degree of water loss from the airways and thus the chance of having EIB. Reducing water loss from the airways decreases the possibility of EIB. On average, air humidity of swimming pools is about 60% (and likely close to full saturation at the surface of the water), whereas mean air temperature is usually around 27°C.[13,30] Inhaling such humid and warm air during swimming can protect against EIB or reduce its magnitude. Although this has been debated,[31] swimming remains less asthmogenic compared with running when minute ventilation and the water content of inspired air during exercise are similar.[22,25] At the same ventilatory rate, when the air is dry and less than 10 mg/H_2O per liter, treadmill running but not swimming generally induces EIB in subjects with asthma.[25]

Influence of Hydrostatic Pressure, Body Immersion, and Breathing Pattern

The hydrostatic pressure exerts compression on the chest, which facilitates expiration,[32] and suppresses the dependence on gravity, facilitating the return of venous blood from the legs to the chest.[33] The shift of blood volume is thought to play a role in modulating heat exchange and EIB.[26] This was demonstrated by Gilbert and colleagues[26] who studied the influence of wearing antishock trousers (which cause blood to shift acutely from the legs to the thorax on the airway response) to 4-minute hyperpnea challenge. Whereas no change in FEV_1 was observed in control subjects after wearing or not wearing antishock trousers (mean posttest FEV_1 fall, 2 ± 1%), in subjects with asthma, a significant reduction of bronchoconstriction was observed (the mean posttest FEV_1 fall was 21% without and 3% with antishock trousers). The authors suggested that the shift of blood from the legs to the thorax attenuated hyperpnea-induced bronchoconstriction because of a concomitant change in airway blood supply, which increases airstream temperature and disrupts thermal gradient that develops after hyperpnea. However, the recumbent position also increases the thoracic venous return yet it provides no protective effect against EIB.[34]

A controlled breathing pattern caused by the different types of swimming, the mouth being frequently under the water surface except in backstroke, and characterized by a prolonged expiration, a short duration of inspiration, and hypoventilation may induce CO_2 retention.[27] The resulting hypercapnia can then induce a bronchodilation protecting from development of EIB.[27]

Swimming Programs in Subjects with Asthma

Few studies have been conducted on the influence of physical activity programs in swimming pools on severity and frequency of asthma exacerbations. Generally, the authors recommend a 2-month physical retraining with 2- or 3-weekly sessions lasting 30 to 45 minutes, preferentially as interval training.[35–42] The intensity of exercise varies from one study to another, but exercising at the load at which ventilation and carbon dioxide increase disproportionately to oxygen uptake (first ventilatory threshold) combined with high-intensity periods has been shown to be well-tolerated for rehabilitating people with respiratory diseases.[37,39] Swimming programs in subjects with asthma lead to an improvement in aerobic capacity, with a concomitant increase in the workload required to provoke EIB, a decrease in the severity of asthma exacerbations,[36,40] hospitalization rate or unscheduled physician visits,[42] daily medication,[36,38] school absenteeism,[40] and improved quality of life.[39,40] Airway responsiveness may be slightly reduced after swimming programs[42] or unchanged.[36,38] The benefits are probably not caused by swimming itself, but rather by the effects of participation in an exercise program, as suggested by studies showing improvements with non-swimming–related training activities.[43] Moreover, there is a possible influence on the airways of an increased cholinergic tone caused by the immersion of the face in cold water (diving reflex).[44] A positive correlation has also been observed between the decrease in heart rate caused by the diving reflex and the dose of methacholine inducing a 45% fall in airway-specific conductance.[44] The increased cholinergic tone observed in asthma may play a role in the bronchoconstriction during face immersion in cold water.[45]

Subjects with asthma who would like to perform swimming activities are often encouraged to do so in a warm and humid environment. Physical activities other than swimming, however, may also be beneficial and could be selected according to subjects' preference. The potential problem of exposure to airborne irritants resulting from water chlorination has not yet been fully addressed and the long-term effects of swimming training programs need to be better documented.[36,40,41] Subjects with asthma often report respiratory symptoms and may develop airway hyperresponsiveness (AHR) after attendance at a chlorinated pool,[46–48] but swimming is less potent than other types of exercises in provoking bronchoconstriction. It should be stressed that most sports are well tolerated when medication is taken for prevention of EIB (although if asthma is well controlled, the athletes rarely need a short-term preventative medication, such as inhaled short-acting β_2 agonists).

EFFECTS OF CHLORINE-DISINFECTED SWIMMING POOL ENVIRONMENT IN CHILDREN AND RECREATIONAL SWIMMERS

The interaction of chlorine with organic material and ammonium introduced into the pool water by bathers, such as sweat, urine, soap residues, and cosmetics, produces a variety of disinfection by-products (DBPs).[30,49] Some DBPs are irritating for the airways, whereas others are suspected of having carcinogenic potential with repeated exposure to high concentrations.[49] The agents most often described as potential inducers of respiratory disorders are gaseous trichloramines (NCl_3). The aerosols of these products, just above the pool water, may also be detrimental but there are few data available on the effects of these compounds.[49–52] The levels of DBPs in the air depend on several parameters, such as the quantity of organic matter brought by bathers into the water, the efficiency of the ventilation, water renewal, and water characteristics.[49]

Chronic Effects

The acute toxicity from inhaling high concentrations of chlorine and its by-products has been recognized for a long time.[53–60] Evidence that low-dose exposure to chlorine products may chronically damage the respiratory tract of elite swimmers, lifeguards, and pool workers is also increasing.[11–21] Whether these products affect recreational swimmers and children regularly attending chlorinated pools is, however, still controversial. A few recent cross-sectional studies involving child and adolescent recreational swimmers or adult swimmers have suggested a relationship between chlorinated swimming pool attendance and the development of asthma or allergic diseases.[5,8–10,61–64] In those attending swimming pools during infancy, a higher risk of bronchiolitis, which increases the risk of asthma and allergic sensitization, has also been suggested,[7,65] although not confirmed.[66] These findings, however, do not allow a conclusion to be made in favor of an association between attendance at swimming pools by recreational swimmers and the development of asthma or allergic diseases. To the contrary, a recent prospective longitudinal study performed in 5738 British children suggested that swimming did not increase the risk of asthma or allergic symptoms.[67] Furthermore, in this last study, swimming was associated with improved lung function and a lower risk of asthma symptoms, especially among children with preexisting respiratory conditions. These controversial data stress the need for further research on the role of swimming pool attendance in the development of allergic diseases and asthma. Importantly, studies should be comparable and use similar inclusion criteria, methodology, and statistical models to avoid inconsistencies. For example, hygiene measures for swimming pool management vary among the countries and can lead to different results.

The "Chlorine Asthma Hypothesis"

Carbonnelle and colleagues[6] described a transient epithelial injury after a 1-hour swimming session in a chlorinated environment in recreational swimmers, children, or passively exposed attendees. As proposed by Bernard,[52] such epithelial injury could allow allergens to easy access to antigen-presenting cells, and possibly promote allergen sensitization (**Fig. 1**). It is possible that the development of allergic diseases and asthma could be facilitated by repeated attendance at chlorinated swimming pools in association with allergen exposure. The time of recovery from the epithelium injury is short (12–24 hours)[6] and it remains to be determined whether recreational swimmers training twice a week or more are at risk of developing allergic diseases or asthma. There is nevertheless a need to improve disinfection techniques and the hygiene and ventilation in indoor swimming pools to minimize chlorine by-product inhalation and allow bathers to swim without significant risk. Further studies should also consider swimming-induced rhinitis in a chlorinated environment, a frequent problem that remains insufficiently studied.

ELITE SWIMMERS' AIRWAYS

Swimmers, including synchronized swimmers, may train more than 30 hours per week, and, if so, they belong to the athletic population with the highest number of annual training hours. Consequently, they are particularly exposed to by-products of chlorine-disinfection, especially NCl_3, which they probably inhale in high concentrations from the air just above the water. It has been suggested that the increased

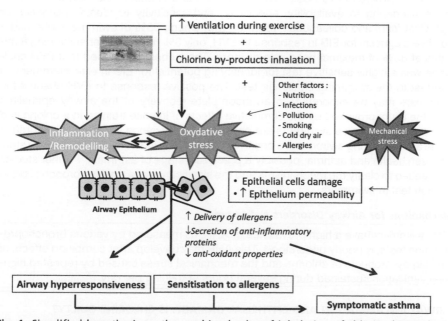

Fig. 1. Simplified hypothesis on the combined roles of inhalation of chlorine by-products and exercise in allergic sensitization, airway hyperresponsiveness, and asthma development. *Bold lines* represent the additional effect of chlorine by-products on exercise. (*Data from* Bernard A. Chlorination products: emerging links with allergic diseases. Curr Med Chem 2007;14:1689–99.)

prevalence of allergy, respiratory symptoms, and AHR in swimmers who compete is caused by the combined effects of DBP inhalation and the many hours per week of training.[11,13,15]

Prevalence of Airway Disorders and EIB in Swimmers

Swimmers are affected by lower and upper respiratory symptoms. During the training season, 74% of competitive swimmers complain of nasal obstruction, rhinorrhea, sneezing, or itching.[68,69] Screening of competitive swimmers has also demonstrated that up to 76% may have AHR or EIB when measured in the laboratory.[11,12] The prevalence of asthma before starting a competitive career seems to be similar or slightly increased in swimmers, compared with athletes performing other sports or healthy subjects. This suggests that most commonly, swimmers do not begin swimming because of asthma, but rather develop respiratory disorders associated with asthma during their athletic career. It is the recreational swimmers or children, rather than the swimmers in training, who complain most often of respiratory symptoms attributed to a strong chemical odor of chlorine.[13,70] Asymptomatic AHR or EIB seems to occur more frequently in swimmers compared with athletes performing other sports,[15] which raises the question of symptom perception in competitive swimmers and the clinical significance of AHR or EIB as documented in a laboratory environment.

Significance of AHR and EIB

Several tests may be performed to diagnose EIB: exercise itself; eucapnic voluntary hyperpnea of dry air (EVH); and inhalation of hyperosmolar aerosols, or mannitol (discussed elsewhere in this issue). The choice of the bronchoprovocation test is often made according to availability, specificity, and sensitivity to identify potential for EIB. Castricum and colleagues[71] reported that among 55% of swimmers who had a positive diagnosis for EIB in response to EVH, only 3% had EIB after swimming 8 minutes at 85% of maximal heart rate or more. The authors concluded that EVH challenge was a highly sensitive test for identifying potential for EIB in elite swimmers, in contrast to the swimming challenge test. The positive response to EVH observed in swimmers may be secondary to an incomplete recovery of the airway epithelium from the injury provoked by the cumulative effects of intense training in a chlorinated environment. Because swimmers are not likely to experience significant dehydration of the airways during swimming, a positive EVH test may indicate an intermediary state between health and asthma, possibly a preclinical stage of asthma.[72] Further studies are needed to clarify the mechanisms and the significance of a positive bronchial provocation test in swimmers.

Mechanisms for Airway Disorders in Swimmers

Why swimmers have a high prevalence of AHR, as measured by various bronchoprovocation tests, is poorly understood. This AHR may develop after combined effects of inhaling by-products of chlorine and the mechanical stress caused by repeated high-level ventilation sustained during several hours of training per day.[73]

AIRWAY INFLAMMATION AND EPITHELIAL DAMAGE: IS CHLORINE GUILTY?

The recent chlorine hypothesis suggests a link between exposure to by-products of chlorine and allergic diseases or asthma in industrialized countries.[52] Inhaled by-products of chlorine have the potential to interact with airway epithelium resulting in oxidative stress and airway inflammation. When inhalation of these by-products occurs repeatedly in elite swimmers it may result in an impairment of antioxidant activity in the airways,[74] and contribute to the development of allergic diseases,[52] increased airway responsiveness,[11–15] or symptomatic asthma.[14,75,76] Inflammatory and remodeling processes have been observed in the bronchial mucosa of competitive swimmers when compared with nonathletes with mild asthma.[76] The structural changes observed in the bronchi of swimmers were independent of the documentation of AHR.[76] We consider from our observations and others that intense swim training in a chlorinated swimming pool on a recurrent basis may promote the development of a specific phenotype of asthmatic airways in elite swimmers.

Despite the evidence implicating inhalation of chlorine by-products in the development of airway disorders, the observed structural changes and hyperresponsiveness may simply reflect a normal adaptive response to intense training. Indeed, remodeling and inflammation of the airways have also been observed in bronchial biopsies of elite skiers.[77] In elite skiers repeated dry air hyperpnea may cause structural changes, and evidence favors a high minute ventilation for inducing epithelial damage as reflected by markers of increased airway permeability.[6,78]

Upper and Lower Airways Interaction

Respiratory symptoms originating from the upper airways are very common in swimmers.[79,80] In a recent study of nasal cytology, Gelardi and colleagues[68] observed nasal inflammation of a neutrophilic type in most symptomatic elite swimmers, and they attributed this to the irritant effect of chlorine. After 30-days using a nose-clip during swimming, nasal symptoms were significantly reduced, particularly in those with neutrophilic inflammation. This finding highlights the role played by the by-products of chlorine on the nasal mucosa, either by inhaled gases or by the chlorinated water directly entering the nose. It is likely that the effects of these by-products are similar on the upper and lower airway epithelium.[81]

Clinical Consequences and Possible Effects on Performance

Rhinitis has been shown to affect the quality of life of swimmers during an intense period of training, and may thus have an impact on performance.[69] Elite swimmers with a diagnosis of asthma perform as well as or even better than those without asthma during competitions.[82] Although the potential for EIB, as documented by a positive response to EVH, is high among swimmers, most competitive swimmers do not report respiratory symptoms to their physician.[15] It has been suggested that they consider symptoms a normal phenomenon caused by intense training or the presence of chlorine, and do not report them because they do not occur during swimming but rather at another time. A positive response to EVH reveals potential for EIB, and EIB may not necessarily occur after a swimming test or session. Some swimmers, however, may have EIB and be asymptomatic when exercising in the pool environment. Observations from a French study showed a significant reduction in airway responsiveness in eight competitive swimmers after the annual swimming pool cleaning compared with before the cleaning.[83] Moreover, in swimmers AHR/EIB and rhinitis can be transient and a partial remission has been observed after a period of rest as short as 2 weeks without swimming **(Fig. 2)**.[69,84] During a 5-year follow-up study, a significant attenuation of airway responsiveness was reported in 26 elite swimmers after cessation of training for at least 3 months, whereas no change was found in those swimmers who were still involved in competitive swimming.[85] Whether inflammation and remodeling of the airways observed during a swimmer's career may be reversible remains to be determined.

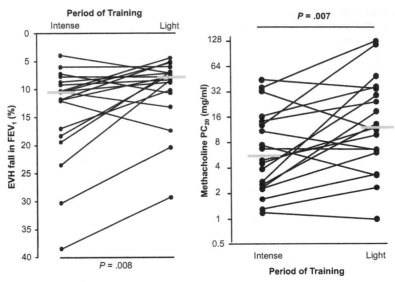

Fig. 2. Individual changes in percentage fall in FEV$_1$ after eucapnic hyperpnea challenge (*left*) and in methacholine PC$_{20}$ (*right*) according to the training period in 19 competitive swimmers. EVH, eucapnic voluntary hyperpnea of dry air. (*Data from* Bougault V, Turmel J, Boulet LP. Airway hyperresponsiveness in elite swimmers: Is it a transient phenomenon? J Allergy Clin Immunol 2011;127:892–8.)

SPECIFIC MANAGEMENT OF AIRWAY DISORDERS AND PREVENTION IN SWIMMERS

Management of asthma in athletes is mainly based on current guideline recommendations,[86,87] and is the same for swimmers as for other athletes. However, whether one should treat asymptomatic swimmers with increased airway responsiveness to a bronchial provocation test as one would for a patient with asthma is still debated and currently difficult to answer. Obviously, the best measure to reduce the potential impact of swimming in chlorinated swimming pools on the airways should be to reduce the release of chlorine by-products into the ambient air of the pool. Because NCl$_3$ levels in the air above swimming pool water are influenced by the interaction between bathers' hygiene and water chlorine by-products, a reduction of human protein matter in the water may lessen respiratory health problems of swimmers. To do so, simple hygienic measures should be taken by the bathers, such as to take a shower and take off make-up and other cosmetics before entering the pool, to wear a swim cap, not to urinate in the water, and to use a swimsuit reserved exclusively for swimming.[88] To reduce exposure to volatile chemical contaminants, the concentration in water should be controlled and there should be adequate air flow across water surface (from forced or natural ventilation) and adequate amounts of fresh air.

One may ask if chlorine disinfection should be replaced by another method. Indeed, alternative chemical disinfectants, such as ozone, copper-silver, and bromine-based products, are being used increasingly. Bromine-based disinfectants are an alternative to chlorination,[89] whereas ozone and ultraviolet irradiation may be useful to eliminate chlorine by-products or reduce the quantity of chlorine required for disinfection.[49,90–92] Copper-silver ionization is also used in some countries and seems to have less deleterious effects on the airways.[9,93] Each disinfectant, however, produces a variety of by-products and has variable efficacy in eliminating microorganisms. The properties of each disinfectant should therefore be assessed more thoroughly to ensure sufficient water disinfection, particularly in high-attendance pools, while avoiding untoward consequences on the airways.

WHAT IS NEXT?

Further studies should be conducted on the specific effects of DBPs on the airways of elite swimmers, and initiated in children and recreational swimmers. The impact of airway disorders on athletic performance and on the health of swimmers during and after their training career should be evaluated. The management of swimming pools can be improved to ensure proper disinfection of the water while also reducing the DBP released. Comparisons of the effects of chlorinated and nonchlorinated swimming pools on the airways and the effects of chlorinated pools with or without the use of strict rules of hygiene should also be promoted.

SUMMARY

Swimming is a healthy activity and is well tolerated by most subjects with asthma. This is likely because of the high humidity of the ambient air that results in less heat and water loss from the airways during exercise reducing the risk of experiencing EIB. For this reason swimming is frequently recommended to subjects with asthma to improve their aerobic capacity and quality of life. However, there is increasing evidence of an impact from exposure to by-products of chlorine on the development of airway disorders, including asthma, AHR, rhinitis, and allergic diseases. Elite swimmers are particularly concerned because the prevalence of airway disorders is the highest among this group compared with other athletes. Both the high ventilation of exercise and the inhalation of chlorine by-products are likely to contribute to the development of these disorders. Further studies are needed to characterize more specifically the role of by-products of chlorine on the airways and the development of the structural changes in the airways that are observed in swimmers.

REFERENCES

1. Bar-Yishay E, Gur I, Inbar O, et al. Difference between swimming and running as stimuli for exercise-induced asthma. Eur J Appl Physiol 1982;48:387–97.
2. Bar-Or O, Inbar O. Swimming and asthma. Sports Med 1992;16:397–405.
3. Piacentini GL, Baraldi E. Pro: swimming in chlorinated pools and risk of asthma: we can now carry on sending our children to swimming pools! Am J Respir Crit Care Med 2011;183:569–70.
4. Bernard A, Voisin C, Sardella A. Con: respiratory risks associated with chlorinated swimming pools: a complex pattern of exposure and effects. Am J Respir Crit Care Med 2011;183:570–2.
5. Bernard A, Nickmilder M, Voicin C, et al. Impact of chlorinated swimming pool attendance on the respiratory health of adolescents. Pediatrics 2009;124:1110–8.
6. Carbonnelle S, Francaux M, Doyle I, et al. Changes in serum pneumoproteins caused by short-term exposures to nitrogen trichloride in indoor chlorinated swimming pools. Biomarkers 2002;7:464–78.
7. Voisin C, Sardella A, Marcucci F, et al. Infant swimming in chlorinated pools and the risks of bronchiolitis, asthma and allergy. Eur Respir J 2010;36:41–7.
8. Bernard A, Nickmilder M, Voisin C. Outdoor swimming pools and the risks of asthma and allergies during adolescence. Eur Respir J 2008;32:979–88.

9. Bernard A, Carbonnelle S, Dumont X, et al. Infant swimming practice, pulmonary epithelium integrity, and the risk of allergic and respiratory diseases later in childhood. Pediatrics 2007;119:1095–103.

10. Chaumont A, Voisin C, Sardella A, et al. Interactions between domestic water hardness, infant swimming and atopy in the development of childhood eczema. Environ Res 2012;116:52–7.

11. Langdeau JB, Turcotte H, Bowie DM, et al. Airway hyperresponsiveness in elite athletes. Am J Respir Crit Care Med 2000;161:1479–84.

12. Zwick H, Popp W, Budik G, et al. Increased sensitization to aeroallergens in competitive swimmers. Lung 1990;168:111–5.

13. Potts JE. Adverse respiratory health effects of competitive swimming: the prevalence of symptoms; illness, and bronchial responsiveness to methacholine and exercise [dissertation]. Vancouver (British Columbia): University of British Columbia; 1994.

14. Helenius IJ, Rytilä P, Metso T, et al. Respiratory symptoms, bronchial responsiveness, and cellular characteristics of induced sputum in elite swimmers. Allergy 1998;53:346–52.

15. Bougault V, Turmel J, Boulet LP. Bronchial challenges and respiratory symptoms in elite swimmers and winter sport athletes: airway hyperresponsiveness in asthma: its measurement and clinical significance. Chest 2010;138:31S–7S.

16. Massin N, Bohadana AB, Wild P, et al. Respiratory symptoms and bronchial responsiveness in lifeguards exposed to nitrogen trichloride in indoor swimming pools. Occup Environ Med 1998;55:258–63.

17. Jacobs JH, Spaan S, van Rooy GB, et al. Exposure to trichloramine and respiratory symptoms in indoor swimming pool workers. Eur Respir J 2007;29:690–8.

18. Nemery B, Hoet PH, Nowak D. Indoor swimming pools, water chlorination and respiratory health. Eur Respir J 2002;19:790–3.

19. Thickett KM, McCoach JS, Gerber JM, et al. Occupational asthma caused by chloramines in indoor swimming-pool air. Eur Respir J 2002;19:827–32.

20. Nordberg GF, Lundstrom NG, Forsberg B, et al. Lung function in volunteers before and after exposure to trichloramine in indoor pool environments and asthma in a cohort of pool workers. BMJ Open 2012;2(5). pii:e000973.

21. Fantuzzi G, Righi E, Predieri G, et al. Airborne trichloramine (NCl(3)) levels and self-reported health symptoms in indoor swimming pool workers: dose-response relationships. J Expo Sci Environ Epidemiol 2012. http://dx.doi.org/10.1038/jes.2012.56.

22. McFadden ER, Gilbert IA. Exercise-induced asthma. N Engl J Med 1994;330:1362–7.

23. Fitch K, Morton AR. Specificity of exercise in exercise-induced asthma. Br Med J 1971;4:577–81.

24. Ram FS, Robinson SM, Black PN, et al. Physical training for asthma. Cochrane Database Syst Rev 2005;(4):CD001116.

25. Inbar O, Dotan R, Dlin RA, et al. Breathing dry or humid air and exercise-induced asthma during swimming. Eur J Appl Physiol 1980;44:43–50.

26. Gilbert IA, Regnard J, Lenner KA, et al. Intrathoracic airstream temperatures during acute expansions of thoracic blood volume. Clin Sci 1991;81:655–61.

27. Donnelly PM. Exercise-induced asthma: the protective role of CO_2 during swimming. Lancet 1991;337:179–80.

28. Bar-Or O, Neuman I, Dotan R. Effects of dry and humid climates on exercise-induced asthma in children and preadolescents. J Allergy Clin Immunol 1977;60:163–8.

29. Anderson SD, Daviskas E. The mechanisms of exercise-induced asthma is.... J Allergy Clin Immunol 2000;106:453–9.
30. Drobnic F, Freixa A, Casan P, et al. Assessment of chlorine exposure in swimmers during training. Med Sci Sports Exerc 1996;28:271–4.
31. Bundgaard A, Schmidt A, Ingemann Hansen T, et al. Exercise-induced asthma after swimming and bicycle exercise. Eur J Respir Dis 1982;63:245–8.
32. Withers RT, Hamdorf PA. Effect of immersion on lung capacities and volumes: implications for the densitometric estimation of relative body fat. J Sports Sci 1989;7:21–30.
33. Park KS, Choi JK, Park YS. Cardiovascular regulation during water immersion. Appl Human Sci 1999;18:233–41.
34. Inbar O, Naiss S, Neuman E, et al. The effect of body posture on exercise- and hyperventilation- induced asthma. Chest 1991;100:1229–34.
35. Emtner M, Herala M, Stalenheim G. High intensity physical training in adults with asthma. Chest 1996;109:323–30.
36. Fitch KD, Morton AR, Blansky BA. Effects of swimming training on children with asthma. Arch Dis Child 1976;51:190–4.
37. Varray A, Mercier JG, Préfaut CG. Individualized training reduces excessive hyperventilation in asthmatics. Int J Rehabil Res 1995;18:297–312.
38. Weisgerber MC, Guill M, Weisgerber JM, et al. Benefits of swimming in asthma: effect of a session of swimming lessons on symptoms and PFTs with review of the literature. J Asthma 2003;40:453–64.
39. Weisgerber M, Webber K, Meurer J, et al. Moderate and vigorous exercise programs in children with asthma: safety, parental satisfaction, and asthma outcomes. Pediatr Pulmonol 2008;43:1175–82.
40. Wardell CP, Isbister C. A swimming program for children with asthma. Does it improve their quality of life? Med J Aust 2000;173:647–8.
41. Matsumoto I, Araki H, Tsuda K, et al. Effects of swimming training on aerobic capacity and exercise-induced bronchoconstriction in children with bronchial asthma. Thorax 1999;54:196–201.
42. Wicher IB, Ribeiro MA, Marmo DB, et al. Effects of swimming on spirometric parameters and bronchial hyperresponsiveness in children and adolescents with moderate persistent atopic asthma. J Pediatr (Rio J) 2010;86:384–90.
43. Chandratilleke MG, Carson KV, Picot J, et al. Physical training for asthma. Cochrane Database Syst Rev 2012;(5):CD001116.
44. Sturani C, Sturani A, Tosi I. Parasympathetic activity assessed by diving-reflex and by airway response to methacholine in bronchial asthma and rhinitis. Respiration 1985;48:321–8.
45. Kallenbach JM, Webster T, Dowdeswell R, et al. Reflex heart rate control in asthma. Evidence of parasympathetic overactivity. Chest 1985;85:644–8.
46. Penny PT. Swimming pool wheezing. Br Med J (Clin Res Ed) 1983;287:461–2.
47. Mustchin CP, Pickering CA. "Coughing water": bronchial hyperreactivity induced by swimming in a chlorinated pool. Thorax 1979;34:682–3.
48. Stav D, Stav M. Asthma and whirlpool baths. N Engl J Med 2005;353:1635–6.
49. World Health Organization. International programme on chemical safety, environmental health criteria 216: disinfectants and disinfectant by-products. Geneva (Switzerland): WHO; 2000.
50. Keuten MG, Schets FM, Schijven JF, et al. Definition and quantification of initial anthropogenic pollutant release in swimming pools. Water Res 2012;46:3682–92.

51. Varraso R, Massin N, Hery M, et al. Not only training but also exposure to chlorinated compounds generates response to oxidative stimuli in swimmers. Toxicol Ind Health 2002;18:269–78.
52. Bernard A. Chlorination products: emerging links with allergic diseases. Curr Med Chem 2007;14:1689–99.
53. Agabiti N, Ancona C, Forastiere F, et al. Short term respiratory effects of acute exposure to chlorine due to a swimming pool accident. Occup Environ Med 2001;58:399–404.
54. Lemiere C, Malo JL, Boutet M. Reactive airways dysfunction syndrome due to chlorine: sequential bronchial biopsies and functional assessment. Eur Respir J 1997;10:241–4.
55. Parimon T, Kanne JP, Pierson DJ. Acute inhalation injury with evidence of diffuse bronchiolitis following chlorine gas exposure at a swimming-pool. Respir Care 2004;49:291–4.
56. Deschamps D, Soler P, Rosenberg N, et al. Persistent asthma after inhalation of a mixture of sodium hypochlorite and hypochloric acid. Chest 1994;105:1895–6.
57. Martinez TT, Long C. Explosion risk from swimming pool chlorinators and review of chlorine toxicity. J Toxicol Clin Toxicol 1995;33:349–54.
58. Bonetto G, Corradi M, Carraro S, et al. Longitudinal monitoring of lung injury in children after acute chlorine exposure in a swimming-pool. Am J Respir Crit Care Med 2006;174:545–9.
59. Ploysongsang Y, Beach BC, DiLisio RE. Pulmonary function changes after acute inhalation of chlorine gas. South Med J 1982;75:23–6.
60. D'Alessandro A, Kuschner W, Wong H, et al. Exaggerated responses to chlorine inhalation among persons with non-specific airway hyperreactivity. Chest 1996;109:331–7.
61. Cotter A, Ryan CA. The pool chlorine hypothesis and asthma among boys. Ir Med J 2009;102:79–82.
62. Kohlhammer Y, Döring A, Schäfer T, et al. Swimming pool attendance and hay fever rates later in life. Allergy 2006;61:1305–9.
63. Font-Ribera L, Kogevinas M, Zock JP, et al. Swimming pool attendance and risk of asthma and allergic symptoms in children. Eur Respir J 2009;34:1304–10.
64. Ferrari M, Schenk K, Mantovani W, et al. Attendance at chlorinated indoor pools and risk of asthma in adult recreational swimmers. J Sci Med Sport 2011;14:184–9.
65. Jacobs JH, Fuertes E, Krop EJ, et al. Swimming Pool attendance and respiratory symptoms and allergies among Dutch children. Occup Environ Med 2012;69:823–30.
66. Schoefer Y, Zutavern A, Brockow I, et al. Health risks of early swimming pool attendance. Int J Hyg Environ Health 2008;211:367–73.
67. Font-Ribera L, Villanueva CM, Nieuwenhuijsen MJ, et al. Swimming pool attendance, asthma, allergies, and lung function in the Avon Longitudinal Study of Parents and Children cohort. Am J Respir Crit Care Med 2011;183:582–8.
68. Gelardi M, Ventura MT, Fiorella R, et al. Allergic and non-allergic rhinitis in swimmers: clinical and cytological aspects. Br J Sports Med 2012;46:54–8.
69. Bougault V, Turmel J, Boulet LP. Effect of intense swimming training on rhinitis in high-level competitive swimmers. Clin Exp Allergy 2010;40:1238–46.
70. Levesque B, Duchesne JF, Gingras S, et al. The determinants of prevalence of health complaints among young competitive swimmers. Int Arch Occup Environ Health 2006;80:32–9.

71. Castricum A, Holzer K, Brukner P, et al. The role of the bronchial provocation challenge tests in the diagnosis of exercise-induced bronchoconstriction in elite swimmers. Br J Sports Med 2010;44:736–40.
72. Boulet LP. Asymptomatic airway hyperresponsiveness: a curiosity or an opportunity to prevent asthma? Am J Respir Crit Care Med 2003;167:371–8.
73. Tschumperlin DJ, Drazen JM. Chronic effects of mechanical force on airways. Annu Rev Physiol 2006;68:563–83.
74. Bougault V, Morissette M, Murray N, et al. Oxidative stress in swimmers' airways [abstract]. Eur Respir J 2010;36(Suppl 54):S582.
75. Bougault V, Turmel J, St Laurent J, et al. Asthma, airway inflammation and epithelial damage in swimmers and cold-air athletes. Eur Respir J 2009;33: 740–6.
76. Bougault V, Loubaki L, Joubert P, et al. Airway remodeling and inflammation in competitive swimmers with and without airway hyperresponsiveness. J Allergy Clin Immunol 2012;129:351–8.
77. Karjalainen EM, Laitinen A, Sue-Chu M, et al. Evidence of airway inflammation and remodeling in ski athletes with and without bronchial hyperresponsiveness to methacholine. Am J Respir Crit Care Med 2000;161:2086–91.
78. Nanson CJ, Burgess JL, Robin M, et al. Exercise alters serum pneumoprotein concentrations. Respir Physiol 2001;127:259–65.
79. Deitmer T, Scheffler R. Nasal physiology in swimmers and swimmers' sinusitis. Acta Otolaryngol 1990;110:286–91.
80. Ondolo C, Aversa S, Passali F, et al. Nasal and lung function in competitive swimmers. Acta Otorhinolaryngol Ital 2009;29:137–43.
81. Clearie KL, Vaidyanathan S, Williamson PA, et al. Effects of chlorine and exercise on the unified airway in adolescent elite Scottish swimmers. Allergy 2010;65: 269–73.
82. Fitch KD. An overview of asthma and airway hyper-responsiveness in Olympic athletes. Br J Sports Med 2012;46:413–6.
83. Simon-Rigaud ML, Eechout C, Bourdin H, et al. Hyperréactivité bronchique et natation. Influence de l'entraînement en atmosphère chlorée. Sci Sports 1997; 12:142–7.
84. Bougault V, Turmel J, Boulet LP. Airway hyperresponsiveness in elite swimmers: Is it a transient phenomenon? J Allergy Clin Immunol 2011;127:892–8.
85. Helenius IJ, Rytila P, Sarna S, et al. Effect of continuing or finishing high-level sports on airway inflammation, bronchial hyperresponsiveness, and asthma. J Allergy Clin Immunol 2002;109:962–8.
86. Anderson SD, Kippelen P. Assessment and prevention of exercise-induced bronchoconstriction. Br J Sports Med 2012;46:391–6.
87. Bonini S, Bonini M, Bousquet J, et al. Rhinitis and asthma in athletes: an ARIA document in collaboration with GA2LEN. Allergy 2006;61:681–92.
88. Bougault V, Boulet LP. Airway dysfunction in swimmers. Br J Sports Med 2012;46: 402–6.
89. Lourencetti C, Grimalt JO, Marco E, et al. Trihalomethanes in chlorine and bromine disinfected swimming pools: air-water distributions and human exposure. Environ Int 2012;15:59–67.
90. Lee J, Jun MJ, Lee MH, et al. Production of various disinfection byproducts in indoor swimming pool waters treated with different disinfection methods. Int J Hyg Environ Health 2010;213:465–74.
91. Wyatt TD, Wilson TS. A bacteriological investigation of two leisure centre swimming pools disinfected with ozone. J Hyg (Lond) 1979;82:425–41.

92. Weng S, Li J, Blatchley ER. Effects of UV 254 irradiation on residual chlorine and DBPs in chlorination of model organic-N precursors in swimming pools. Water Res 2012;46:2674–82.
93. Landeen LK, Yahya MT, Gerba CP. Efficacy of copper and silver ions and reduced levels of free chlorine in inactivation of legionella pneumophila. Appl Environ Microbiol 1989;55:3040–50.

Air Quality and Exercise-Induced Bronchoconstriction in Elite Athletes

Kenneth W. Rundell, PhD[a,b,*], Malcolm Sue-Chu, MB ChB, PhD[c,d]

KEYWORDS

- Air pollution • Cold air • Dry air • Exercise • Breathing • Asthma • Airway damage
- Athlete

KEY POINTS

- The requisite warming and humidification of the inspired air at high ventilation rates can result in airway drying and subsequent damage, inflammation, and bronchial hyperresponsiveness.
- Data from bronchial challenge test studies on the ice-rink athlete show consistently high rates of exercise-induced bronchoconstriction, and recent evidence implicates inhalation of airborne fine and ultrafine particles emitted in the exhaust of fossil-fueled ice-resurfacing machines.
- Replacement of fossil-fuelled resurfacing equipment with electric ice-resurfacing equipment in indoor ice arenas would decrease the level of harmful pollutants.

INTRODUCTION

Aerobic exercise results in cardiovascular changes that support improved health and longevity. However, exercise in cold/dry air or in polluted environments can cause airway injury and airway hyperresponsiveness (AHR), and may lead to the development of asthma. Winter sports athletes compete in both outdoor and indoor environments in conditions that may be harmful to the airways. However, for these athletes, training is a year-round activity and depending on the training venue, exposure may be continuous. The outdoor winter athlete is exposed to the cold/dry air

Funding Sources: No current funding.
Conflict of Interest: Previous Consultant for Merck, Inc. Current Consultant for Pharmaxis Inc (K.W. Rundell). None (M. Sue-Chu).
[a] Pharmaxis Inc, Philadelphia, PA 19341, USA; [b] Commonwealth Medical College, Scranton, PA 18509, USA; [c] Department of Thoracic Medicine, St Olavs Hospital, Trondheim University Hospital, Postbox 3250 Sluppen, NO-7006 Trondheim, Norway; [d] Department of Circulation and Medical Imaging, Institute of Circulation and Imaging, Norwegian University of Science and Technology, Trondheim, Norway
* Corresponding author. Medical Affairs, One East Uwchlan Avenue, Suite 405, Exton, PA 19341.
E-mail address: Ken.rundell@pharmaxis.com

during the competitive season and may also be exposed to traffic-related pollutants and ozone during off-season training, depending on the athlete's training location. The ice-rink athlete could be exposed to high pollutants emitted from ice-resurfacing machines as well as to cold/dry air throughout the competitive and noncompetitive seasons.

Exercise-induced bronchoconstriction (EIB) is the transient narrowing of the airways usually occurring within 20 minutes after exercise, but can occur during the exercise, and spontaneously resolves within 30 to 60 minutes. Theories for pathogenesis of EIB include the hyperosmolar hypothesis, which postulates hyperpnea-induced drying of the airways with subsequent increase in cell osmolarity and release of bronchoconstricting mediators from inflammatory cells.[1] The airway-cooling hypothesis is based on a reduction of intra-airway temperature during exercise and development of a reactive hyperemia after exercise in response to airway cooling.[2] Smooth-muscle contraction in response to inflammatory mediators and a reduction in airway caliber from hyperemia have been suggested to be responsible for EIB.[3] However, EIB is not a universal response to exercise in all athletes, and other factors such as environmental and personal risk factors are involved in determining the response.[4] Environmental factors, such as quality, relative humidity, and temperature of the inspired air during training and competition, affect all athletes, while allergens are of importance in atopic athletes. On an individual level, factors such as the response of the parasympathetic nervous system, the degree of neurogenic-mediated immune inflammation, and genetic susceptibility may be significant. However, the interaction between environmental and personal risk factors may determine the response of the airway to strenuous exercise.[4]

EFFECT OF COLD AIR

Cold air can serve as a more severe stimulus to the airway, primarily because the air is dry, even when fully saturated with water vapor. The relationship between the water-vapor content in air at a given relative humidity and temperature is curvilinear (**Fig. 1**).[5] At an ambient temperature of $-10°$, $0°$, $+10°$, and $37°C$ the maximum water content is 3, 5, 9, and 44 mg/L, respectively. Thus, conditioning of air from $-10°C$ to body temperature requires the addition of 41 mg of water per liter of air, and causes a decrease in intra-airway temperature. At a ventilation rate of 60 L/min for 4 minutes, the decrease in temperature is $4°C$ greater when breathing air at $-17°C$, in comparison with air at room temperature.[6] Expiratory water losses and, thus, dehydration of the airways will be greater during training/competition at lower ambient temperatures. The long-term effects of exercise in cold/dry air have not been investigated in longitudinal studies in human winter-sports athletes. Most studies evaluating the prevalence of EIB in both winter and summer athletes are cross-sectional in design and report on a specific sport population with a typically small number of subjects. However, a decrease of lung function has been observed in 3 cross-country skiers followed over a period of 9 to 12 years.[7] In addition, the prevalence of respiratory symptoms and AHR to direct stimuli is increased together with evidence of airway inflammation and remodeling in cross-sectional studies.[7–9] Neutrophilic inflammation in the submucosa with lymphocyte aggregates is seen in bronchial biopsies in cross-country skiers,[8,9] whereas increased counts of neutrophils and, to a lesser degree, of eosinophils are present in induced sputum in ice hockey players.[10]

EFFECT OF AIRBORNE POLLUTION

Exercise in environments containing high levels of respirable pollutants has both acute and chronic effects on the airways and the cardiovascular system; this is of special

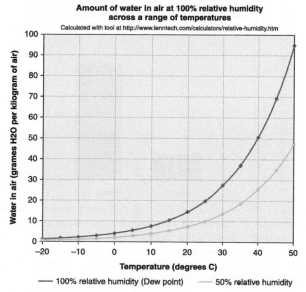

Fig. 1. Curvilinear relationship between water content in air and ambient temperature.

interest to elite athletes because of the high ventilations they achieve and sustain during exercise.[11–13] The serious athlete may be at greater risk to these environmental influences than the recreational athlete because of the greater overall exposure and increased deposition of pollutants from the high training volumes at increased minute ventilation. Ultrafine particles (UPM, particles <100 nm diameter; **Fig. 2**), those that are emitted in high concentrations from internal combustion engines, have greater deposition efficiency than larger particles,[11,12] are highly oxidative,[14] and induce pulmonary inflammation (**Fig. 3**).[15–19]

A causative relationship between exposure to air pollution and the development of asthma, AHR, and increased asthma exacerbations is supported by several

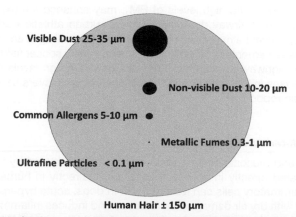

Fig. 2. Size relationship between ultrafine particles, metallic fumes, common allergens, non-visible dust, and visible dust within a cross section of a human hair.

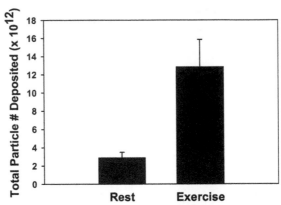

Fig. 3. Total number of deposited particles during rest and 1 hour of moderate exercise at 38 ± 9.5 L/min ventilation. Deposition of particles of 26 ± 1.6 nm diameter during exercise was found to be more than 4.5-fold higher than at rest because of the increase in deposition fraction of the smaller particles coupled with increased minute ventilation. (*Redrawn from* Daigle CC, Chalupa DC, Gibb FR, et al. Ultrafine particle deposition in humans during rest and exercise. Inhal Toxicol 2003;15(6):539–52.)

studies.[20–26] Urban and occupational air quality has recently received much attention, although few studies specifically address the consequence of exercise in high-particulate ambient air environments. Several emission-related airborne pollutants have been identified as harmful: ozone (O_3), sulfur dioxide (SO_2), nitrogen oxides (NO_x) and particulate matter ($PM_{2.5}$, particles <2.5 μm diameter). Ozone, nitrogen dioxide, and freshly generated particulate matter (PM) from internal combustion engines are the primary pollutants of concern in the outdoor environment, although indoor air quality (AQ) is of importance; trichloramine (NCl_3), a gas formed in chlorinated pools, has been implicated in swimmer asthma.[27]

Investigators have examined the relationship between ice-rink AQ[28] and EIB, and have associated the high prevalence of EIB identified in skating athletes to inhalation of PM_1 (PM <1 μm diameter).[21–23] The 20% to 50% prevalence of EIB reported in skaters[21,22,29,30] is much higher than the estimated 8% to 10% prevalence of asthma in the United States. Chronic ventilation of cold/dry air during sport training and competition, combined with high levels of PM_1, may enhance the expression of, or directly cause, EIB and airway damage. Likewise, urban athletic fields and school playgrounds may present a major health concern affecting all ages and genders. Multiple (62 days) measurements of air pollutants at a university soccer field in close proximity to a major highway have shown PM_1 at extremely high levels (**Fig. 4**),[24] and significant decreases in lung function in the college soccer players using these fields has recently been reported.[31]

MECHANISMS
Cold/Dry Air-Induced Airway Injury

Epithelial injury and mucosal inflammation in the airways caused by hyperpnea has been demonstrated directly in animal studies and indirectly in human studies; the presence of inflammatory cells can lead to AHR. In dogs, acute hyperpnea of the peripheral airways with dry air damages the mucosa and induces inflammatory changes and microvascular leakage that persists for more than 24 hours.[32,33] When hyperpnea is repeated over a 4-day period, mucosal edema develops, and is followed by repair of

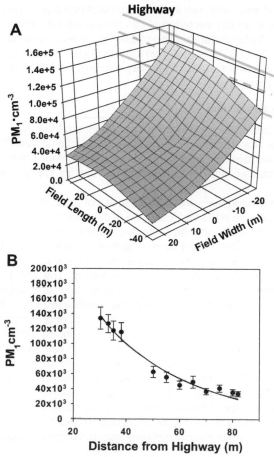

Fig. 4. (*A*) A 3-dimensional blanket graph of the mean values for 62 days at 12 locations at a soccer field located next to a high-traffic roadway shows the increased count at the locations nearest the roadway, with the lower counts furthest away from the roadway. (*B*) The decline in number count moving away from the roadway follows a curvilinear order ($r = -0.99$) and is due to dispersion and particle agglomeration. (*Redrawn from* Rundell KW, Caviston R, Hollenbach AM, et al. Vehicular air pollution, playgrounds, and youth athletic fields. Inhal Toxicol 2006;18(8):541–7.)

the epithelial damage and restoration of normal morphology within 1 week.[34] Similar changes are seen in the bronchiolar epithelial turnover without inflammation in mice, after endurance training at low to moderate intensity at room temperature over 45 days.[35] At 24 to 48 hours after completion of an 1100-mile endurance race in subfreezing conditions there is, in addition to mucosal edema, accumulation of intraluminal debris and an increase of inflammatory cells in the bronchoalveolar lavage (BAL) fluid in racing sled dogs.[36] Furthermore, when horses were exercised at 4°C in comparison with exercise at 25°C,[37] an increased number of ciliated epithelial cells was present in BAL fluid and a local preferential upregulation of the T-helper type 2 cytokines interleukin (IL)-4, IL-5, and IL-10, as well as cytokines IL-2 and IL-6, was noted.[38]

Clara cell protein 16 (CC16) is a protein secreted by Clara cells localized predominantly in the bronchioli, and has an anti-inflammatory function. Increased levels of this protein in the blood and urine may indicate epithelial damage.[39] Recent studies have shown an increase in urinary excretion of this protein after 8 minutes of hyperpnea of dry air,[40] and also after a similar duration of exercise at near maximal aerobic capacity breathing cold dry (4°C, 37% relative humidity) and warm humid (25°C, 94% relative humidity) air. Of note, the increase in urinary excretion of CC16 was blunted by the inhalation of warm humid air.[41]

Pollution-Induced Airway Injury

Many toxicologic pathways have been proposed in establishing the mechanism for pollution-related airway damage. Evidence for airway inflammation[26,42–45] and oxidative stress[46–49] have been identified after both PM exposure and ozone exposure. Likewise, several studies have shown that high particulate loads increase bronchiolar fibrosis.[50–52]

McCreanor and colleagues[26] identified markers of inflammation and reductions in forced expiratory volume in the first 1 second of exhalation (FEV_1) and forced vital capacity (FVC) in 60 mild and moderate asthmatic patients after walking for 2 hours along a London street or in a park. Reductions of up to 6.1% in FEV_1 and 5.4% in FVC after walking on the street were significantly larger than after walking in the park ($P = .04$ and $P = .01$), with $P<.005$ at some time points (**Fig. 5**). The effects were greater for the moderate asthmatics than for the mild asthmatics, and these changes were accompanied by increases in sputum myeloperoxidase (MPO), a marker of neutrophilic inflammation: 24.5 ng/mL and 4.24 ng/mL for street and park walking, respectively. These changes were associated with exposure to ultrafine particles and elemental carbon. Likewise, Salvi and colleagues[53] showed increased neutrophils, mast cells, $CD4^+$ and $CD8^+$ T lymphocytes, and upregulation of the endothelial adhesion molecules intercellular adhesion molecule 1 and vascular cell adhesion molecule 1 in bronchial tissue after exposure to diesel exhaust. Increased sputum neutrophils and MPO were noted after 4 hours of controlled exposure to diesel exhaust without changes in inflammatory markers in peripheral blood.[54] These studies support increased neutrophilic inflammatory pathway from pollution exposure that is localized to the airways.

Reactive oxidants, produced in response to the inhalation of air pollutants, can stress the airway antioxidant system and subsequently harm cellular components, control the expression of genes, and lead to airway inflammation and airway hyperreactivity. In a cohort of 1610 schoolchildren, Islam and colleagues[49] evaluated the effects of genetic variants of glutathione S-transferase (GST) and exercise in high ozone. GST is expressed in the lungs and is essential for glutathione homeostasis, which provides protection from by-products of oxidative stress. An increased risk of asthma development was identified from ozone exposure in individuals with the functional sequence variant in GSTP1 single-nucleotide polymorphism (SNP) at codon 105 (Ile105 homozygotes).[49] This study suggests a strong relationship between airway oxidative stress and the development and severity of asthma. Ercan and colleagues[55] genotyped a total of 196 children with mild asthma, 116 children with moderate to severe asthma, and 255 controls for GST variants. Systemic malondialdehyde (MDA, a marker of lipid peroxidation) increased, and reduced glutathione (GSH) decreased, in mild to severe asthmatics compared with healthy controls ($P<.001$). Further, regression analysis identified asthma and asthma severity associated with oxidative stress. The GSTP1 Ile105 homozygote was more frequent among asthmatics, whereas the GSTP1 Val105 homozygote was less frequent and was associated with asthma severity.[55] The GSTP1 Ile105 homozygote has been associated with an increased risk of asthma in children who participated in outdoor sports in

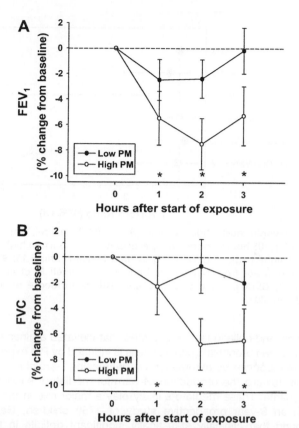

Fig. 5. Sixty adults with mild or moderate asthma were exposed to low ambient particulate matter (PM) and high ambient PM on randomized separate days by walking for 2 hours in each condition. Lung function was measured at 1, 2, 3, 5, 7, and 22 hours from the beginning of the walk. Percent change in forced expiratory volume in 1 second (FEV$_1$) and forced vital capacity (FVC) from baseline values for the first 3 hours are depicted in (A) and (B), respectively. Change in FEV$_1$ was significantly lower for the first 7 hours ($P<.05$), and FVC was significantly lower for the first 3 hours from baseline. (*Redrawn from* McCreanor J, Cullinan P, Nieuwenhuijsen MJ, et al. Respiratory effects of exposure to diesel traffic in persons with asthma. N Engl J Med 2007;357(23):2348–58.)

high-ozone communities (**Fig. 6**).[49] Zaman and colleagues[56] found that S-nitrosoglutathione (GSNO) is formed by the reactions of GSH with nitric oxide in the presence of oxygen, and acts as a potent bronchodilator and aids in cilia motion. Low levels of GSNO, found in asthmatics and patients with cystic fibrosis with chronically low GSH, could be the result of air-pollution–related GSH depletion. It has been shown that low levels of GSNO (0.5–1 μM) increase 5-lipoxygenase (5-LO, an important enzyme in the cysteinyl leukotriene pathway) activity to 6-fold, whereas GSNO levels greater than 5 μM inhibit 5-LO activity and leukotriene (LT) generation.[56] This observation provides an explanation for the predominately LT-driven AHR reported in ice hockey players who are exposed to ice-resurfacing machine exhaust fumes[23] as well as the high urinary levels of LT E$_4$ in asthmatics exposed to fine PM.[57] These findings highlight the importance of the airway antioxidant system as well as the genetic influence of environmental exposure and risk in the development of asthma.

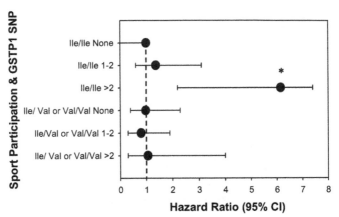

Fig. 6. Using a 2–single nucleotide polymorphism (SNP) model, the Glutathione-*S*-transferase (GST) P1 Ile105 homozygotes who participated in 3 sports in high ozone communities showed the highest risk of developing asthma (hazard ratio 6.15; 95% confidence interval [CI] 2.2–7.4). (*Data from* Islam T, Berhane K, McConnell R, et al. Glutathione-S-transferase (GST) P1, GSTM1, exercise, ozone and asthma incidence in school children. Thorax 2008;64(3):197–202.)

Recently, Hyseni and colleagues[58] suggested that elevated arginase II activity and its expression in human bronchial epithelial cells is induced by PM exposure, and may play a role in the response by asthmatics by decreasing L-arginine concentrations, leading to a shift toward the production of harmful mediators such as superoxide ions and peroxynitrite. These mediators likely play a major role in the pathogenesis of asthma.[59] In an 8-year prospective study of 1759 children, Gauderman and colleagues[20] found that clinically statistically significant deficits in the growth of FEV_1 were associated with nitrogen dioxide ($P = .005$), acid vapor ($P = .004$), $PM_{2.5}$ ($P = .04$), and elemental carbon ($P = .007$). PM exposure can directly induce expression of genes involved in airway-wall fibrosis through nuclear factor κB–mediated and transforming growth factor β–mediated mechanisms, and may play a major role in the airway obstruction observed in individuals chronically exposed to high PM.[60]

PREVALENCE OF AIRWAY DYSFUNCTION IN WINTER ATHLETES

The precise cause of the high prevalence of EIB[22,29,30,61] in winter athletes is unique to the respective training and competition environments. The outdoor winter athlete is exposed to cold/dry air at repeated high minute ventilations during winter sports competition and training. The prevalence of EIB in Nordic skiers has been reported to be 25% to 50%.[62–64] One study found as many as 78% of elite cross-country skiers having symptoms and/or hyperresponsive airways.[65] A more recent study of 46 elite Swedish Nordic skiers reported a lower prevalence of 17% for AHR.[66]

The prevalence of EIB in cold-weather athletes is much higher than the 4% to 15% estimated for the nonathlete population or for the warm-weather athlete.[61,67,68] For the 1998 US Winter Olympic Team, 50% of the Nordic skiers, 43% of the speed skaters, 21% of the figure skaters, 17% of the Nordic combined team, 15% of the ice hockey players, and 9% of the long-track speed skaters had confirmed EIB and/or asthma.[61] The confined space of indoor ice arenas and multiple ice-resurfacing by gas- or propane-powered machines presents significant health risks to the skating athlete. The high prevalence of EIB in skaters[10,21,22,29,30,61,69] and the documented high levels of PM[28] provide evidence for a causal relationship for EIB and decline in resting lung function. High ventilation rates achieved during training and competition will enhance PM deposition efficiency in the lung, making this athlete population especially suscep-tible to effects of PM exposure. These indoor competitors experience a greater prev-alence of EIB, more asthma-like symptoms, and a greater degree of small-airway dysfunction than do outdoor winter athletes.[10,21,22,69] A large percentage of ice-arena athletes who have low resting pulmonary function consistent with chronic small-airway inflammation have been identified.[21,22] Rundell and colleagues[22] found that 39.5% of elite women hockey players presented symptoms of asthma and 21% demonstrated EIB, while Lumme and colleagues[10] found that 52% of elite Finnish hockey players reported symptoms and 24% had bronchial hyperresponsive-ness (BHR) to a histamine challenge. Considering that ice-arena athletes train under conditions whereby ambient temperature and humidity are not as extreme as for their outdoor counterparts, this finding seems paradoxic to the hypothesis that EIB in winter athletes is caused by thermal damage to the airways.[70]

In swimmers, chloramines above the water may trigger EIB and likely generate oxidative stress in the airways. Swimmers with longer duration of exposure tend to have a higher prevalence of EIB.[27,71,72] In a 5-year prospective follow-up study, a decreased incidence of EIB and airway inflammation was observed after discontinu-ation of swimming by elite swimmers.[73] Castricum and colleagues[74] evaluated 33 elite swimmers undergoing eucapnic voluntary hyperpnea (EVH), an 8-minute swim chal-lenge, and an 8-minute laboratory cycle challenge in ambient air. Thirty-nine percent had a clinical diagnosis of asthma and 55%, 3%, and 12% tested positive by EVH, swim test, and cycle test, respectively.

SUMMARY

A true prevalence of EIB in elite winter athletes is difficult to obtain because of incon-sistencies in the way a diagnosis is made. Some studies have used direct challenge tests, others have used a variety of indirect bronchial challenge tests, and others have relied on questionnaires or self-reported symptoms. The outdoor winter athlete typically trains and competes in a cold environment where air water content is quite low. The requisite warming and humidification of the inspired air at high ventilation rates can result in airway drying and subsequent damage, inflammation, and BHR. Data from bronchial challenge test studies on the ice-rink athlete show consistently high rates of EIB, and recent evidence implicates inhalation of airborne fine and ultra-fine particles emitted in the exhaust of fossil-fueled ice-resurfacing machines. Not only are these athletes at risk, but those who train in the urban environment where pollution is high are also at potential risk for airway damage. Likewise, inhalation of airborne Teflon particles from fluorinated waxes in the confines of the waxing room may be an added risk to the skier. Several studies have shown evidence of high oxidative stress, airway inflammation, and airway remodeling related to particle inhalation. Although swimmers are not winter athletes per se, the serious swimmer is exposed to high concentrations of trichloramines at the pool-surface level all the year round. Trichloramine is highly oxidative and has been linked to asthma and EIB in swimmers, and this is discussed in the article by Bougault and Boulet elsewhere in this issue. The harsh conditions endured by the outdoor winter athlete cannot be changed. However, the use of a heat-exchanger mask has been shown to be as effective as pretreatment albuterol[75] in blocking the EIB response, and could be used in training when condi-tions are extremely cold. It has also been suggested that training through mild respiratory infections places the airways at additional risk for damage, and should not be done. Replacement of fossil-fueled resurfacing equipment with electric ice-resurfacing equipment in indoor ice arenas would decrease the level of harmful pollutants. For the athlete who trains in the urban environment, it would be wise to design training routes around low-traffic hours and in low-traffic areas. Of course the athlete will not be able to avoid all hazardous conditions, but an attempt to minimize exposure could have a beneficial and significant effect.

REFERENCES

1. Anderson SD. Is there a unifying hypothesis for exercise-induced asthma? J Allergy Clin Immunol 1984;73:660–5.
2. McFadden ER. Hypothesis: exercise-induced asthma as a vascular phenomenon. Lancet 1990;1:880–3.
3. Anderson SD, Kippelen P. Exercise-induced bronchoconstriction: pathogenesis. Curr Allergy Asthma Rep 2005;5:116–22.
4. Moreira A, Delgado L, Carlsen KH. Exercise-induced asthma: why is it so frequent in Olympic athletes? Expert Rev Respir Med 2011;5:1–3.
5. Available at: http://en.wikipedia.org/wiki/Relative_humidity. Accessed December 12, 2012.
6. McFadden ER Jr, Denison DM, Waller JF, et al. Direct recordings of the temperatures in the tracheobronchial tree in normal man. J Clin Invest 1982;69:700–5.
7. Vergès S, Flore P, Blanchi MP, et al. A 10-year follow-up study of pulmonary function in symptomatic elite cross-country skiers—athletes and bronchial dysfunctions. Scand J Med Sci Sports 2004;14:381–7.
8. Karjalainen EM, Laitinen A, Sue-Chu M, et al. Evidence of airway inflammation and remodeling in ski athletes with and without bronchial hyperresponsiveness to methacholine. Am J Respir Crit Care Med 2000;161:2086–91.
9. Sue-Chu M, Karjalainen EM, Altraja A, et al. Lymphoid aggregates in endobronchial biopsies from young elite cross-country skiers. Am J Respir Crit Care Med 1998;158:597–601.
10. Lumme A, Haahtela T, Ounap J, et al. Airway inflammation, bronchial hyperresponsiveness and asthma in elite ice hockey players. Eur Respir J 2003;22:113–7.
11. Daigle CC, Chalupa DC, Gibb FR, et al. Ultrafine particle deposition in humans during rest and exercise. Inhal Toxicol 2003;15(6):539–52.
12. Chalupa DC, Morrow PE, Oberdörster G, et al. Ultrafine particle deposition in subjects with asthma. Environ Health Perspect 2004;112(8):879–82.
13. Oravisjärvi K, Pietikäinen M, Ruuskanen J, et al. Effects of physical activity on the deposition of traffic-related particles into the human lungs in silico. Sci Total Environ 2011;409(21):4511–8.
14. Li N, Hao M, Phalen RF, et al. Particulate air pollutants and asthma. A paradigm for the role of oxidative stress in PM-induced adverse health effects. Clin Immunol 2003;109(3):250–65.
15. Campen MJ, Lund A, Rosenfeld M. Mechanisms linking traffic-related air pollution and atherosclerosis. Curr Opin Pulm Med 2012;18(2):155–60.
16. Frampton MW, Utell MJ, Zareba W, et al. Effects of exposure to ultrafine carbon particles in healthy subjects and subjects with asthma. Res Rep Health Eff Inst 2004;126:1–47.
17. Huang YC, Rappold AG, Graff DW, et al. Synergistic effects of exposure to concentrated ambient fine pollution particles and nitrogen dioxide in humans. Inhal Toxicol 2012;24(12):790–7.

18. Li XY, Brown D, Smith S, et al. Short-term inflammatory responses following intra-tracheal instillation of fine and ultrafine carbon black in rats. Inhal Toxicol 1999; 11(8):709–31.
19. Oberdörster G, Ferin J, Lehnert BE. Correlation between particle size, in vivo particle persistence, and lung injury. Environ Health Perspect 1994;102(Suppl 5): 173–9.
20. Gauderman WJ, Avol E, Gilliland F, et al. The effect of air pollution on lung development from 10 to 18 years of age. N Engl J Med 2004;351(11):1057–67.
21. Rundell KW. Pulmonary function decay in women ice hockey players: is there a relationship to ice rink air quality? Inhal Toxicol 2004;16(3):117–23.
22. Rundell KW, Spiering BA, Evans TM, et al. Baseline lung function, exercise-induced bronchoconstriction, and asthma-like symptoms in elite women ice hockey players. Med Sci Sports Exerc 2004;36(3):405–10.
23. Rundell KW, Spiering BA, Baumann JM, et al. Bronchoconstriction provoked by exercise in a high-particulate-matter environment is attenuated by montelukast. Inhal Toxicol 2005;17(2):99–105.
24. Rundell KW, Caviston R, Hollenbach AM, et al. Vehicular air pollution, playgrounds, and youth athletic fields. Inhal Toxicol 2006;18(8):541–7.
25. Schwartz J, Neas LM. Fine particles are more strongly associated than coarse particles with acute respiratory health effects in schoolchildren. Epidemiology 2000;11(1):6–10.
26. McCreanor J, Cullinan P, Nieuwenhuijsen MJ, et al. Respiratory effects of exposure to diesel traffic in persons with asthma. N Engl J Med 2007;357(23):2348–58.
27. Bernard A. Chlorination products: emerging links with allergic diseases. Curr Med Chem 2007;14(16):1771–82.
28. Rundell KW. High levels of airborne ultrafine and fine particulate matter in indoor ice arenas. Inhal Toxicol 2003;15(3):237–50.
29. Mannix ET, Farber MO, Palange P, et al. Exercise-induced asthma in figure skaters. Chest 1996;109(2):312–5.
30. Provost-Craig MA, Arbour KS, Sestili DC, et al. The incidence of exercise-induced bronchospasm in competitive figure skaters. J Asthma 1996;33(1):67–71.
31. Hollenbach AM, Caviston R, Rundell KW. Exercise while breathing high ambient auto/truck emission causes decreased lung function in non-asthmatic subjects. Med Sci Sports Exerc 2007;39(5):S323.
32. Freed AN, Omori C, Schofield BH, et al. Dry air-induced mucosal cell injury and bronchovascular leakage in canine peripheral airways. Am J Respir Cell Mol Biol 1994;11:724–32.
33. Omori C, Schofield BH, Mitzner W, et al. Hyperpnea with dry air causes time-dependent alterations in mucosal morphology and bronchovascular permeability. J Appl Physiol 1995;78(3):1043–105.
34. Davis MS, Schofi eld B, Freed AN. Repeated peripheral airway hyperpnea causes inflammation and remodeling in dogs. Med Sci Sports Exerc 2003;35:608–16.
35. Chimenti L, Morici G, Paternò A, et al. Endurance training damages small airway epithelium in mice. Am J Respir Crit Care Med 2007;175(5):442–9.
36. Davis MS, McKiernan B, McCullough S, et al. Racing Alaskan sled dogs as a model of "ski asthma". Am J Respir Crit Care Med 2002;166:878–82.
37. Davis MS, Williams CC, Meinkoth JH, et al. Influx of neutrophils and persistence of cytokine expression in airways of horses after performing exercise while breathing cold air. Am J Vet Res 2007;68:185–9.
38. Davis MS, Malayer JR, Vandeventer L, et al. Cold weather exercise and airway cytokine expression. J Appl Physiol 2005;98:2132–6.

39. Broeckaert F, Arsalane K, Hermans C, et al. Serum Clara cell protein: a sensitive biomarker of increased lung epithelium permeability caused by ambient ozone. Environ Health Perspect 2000;108:533–7.

40. Bolger C, Tufvesson E, Sue-Chu M, et al. Hyperpnoea-induced bronchoconstriction and urinary CC16 levels in athletes. Med Sci Sports Exerc 2000;43:1207–13.

41. Bolger C, Tufvesson E, Anderson SD, et al. Effect of inspired air conditions on exercise-induced bronchoconstriction and urinary CC16 levels in athletes. J Appl Physiol 2011;111:1059–65.

42. Barraza-Villarreal A, Sunyer J, Hernandez-Cadena L, et al. Air pollution, airway inflammation, and lung function in a cohort study of Mexico City schoolchildren. Environ Health Perspect 2008;116(6):832–8.

43. Cho WS, Choi M, Han BS, et al. Inflammatory mediators induced by intratracheal instillation of ultrafine amorphous silica particles. Toxicol Lett 2007;175(1–3): 24–33.

44. Donaldson K, Tran CL. Inflammation caused by particles and fibers. Inhal Toxicol 2002;14(1):5–27.

45. Larsson BM, Sehlstedt M, Grunewald J, et al. Road tunnel air pollution induces bronchoalveolar inflammation in healthy subjects. Eur Respir J 2007;29(4):699–705.

46. Rundell KW, Slee JB, Caviston R, et al. Decreased lung function after inhalation of ultrafine and fine particulate matter during exercise is related to decreased total nitrate in exhaled breath condensate. Inhal Toxicol 2008;20(1):1–9.

47. Zielinski H, Mudway IS, Bérubé KA, et al. Modeling the interactions of particulates with epithelial lining fluid antioxidants. Am J Physiol 1999;277:L719–26.

48. Al-Humadi NH, Siegel PD, Lewis DM, et al. Alteration of intracellular cysteine and glutathione levels in alveolar macrophages and lymphocytes by diesel exhaust particle exposure. Environ Health Perspect 2002;110(4):349–53.

49. Islam T, Berhane K, McConnell R, et al. Glutathione-S-transferase (GST) P1, GSTM1, exercise, ozone and asthma incidence in school children. Thorax 2009;64(3):197–202.

50. Souza MB, Saldiva PH, Pope CA 3rd, et al. Respiratory changes due to long-term exposure to urban levels of air pollution: a histopathologic study in humans. Chest 1998;113(5):1312–8.

51. Pinkerton KE, Green FH, Saiki C, et al. Distribution of particulate matter and tissue remodeling in the human lung. Environ Health Perspect 2000;108(11):1063–9.

52. Calderón-Garcidueñas L, Mora-Tiscareño A, Fordham LA, et al. Respiratory damage in children exposed to urban pollution. Pediatr Pulmonol 2003;36(2):148–61.

53. Salvi S, Blomberg A, Rudell B, et al. Acute inflammatory responses in the airways and peripheral blood after short-term exposure to diesel exhaust in healthy human volunteers. Am J Respir Crit Care Med 1999;159(3):702–9.

54. Nightingale JA, Maggs R, Cullinan P, et al. Airway inflammation after controlled exposure to diesel exhaust particulates. Am J Respir Crit Care Med 2000;162(1): 161–6.

55. Ercan H, Birben E, Dizdar EA, et al. Oxidative stress and genetic and epidemiologic determinants of oxidant injury in childhood asthma. J Allergy Clin Immunol 2006;118(5):1097–104.

56. Zaman K, Hanigan MH, Smith A, et al. Endogenous S-nitrosoglutathione modifies 5-lipoxygenase expression in airway epithelial cells. Am J Respir Cell Mol Biol 2006;34(4):387–93.

57. Rabinovitch N, Strand M, Gelfand EW. Particulate levels are associated with early asthma worsening in children with persistent disease. Am J Respir Crit Care Med 2006;173(10):1098–105.

58. Hyseni X, Soukup JM, Huang YC. Pollutant particles induce arginase II in human bronchial epithelial cells. J Toxicol Environ Health A 2012;75(11):624–36.
59. Meurs H, Maarsingh H, Zaagsma J. Arginase and asthma: novel insights into nitric oxide homeostasis and airway hyperresponsiveness. Trends Pharmacol Sci 2003;24(9):450–5.
60. Dai J, Xie C, Vincent R, et al. Air pollution particles produce airway wall remodeling in rat tracheal explants. Am J Respir Cell Mol Biol 2003;29(3 Pt 1):352–8.
61. Wilber RL, Rundell KW, Szmedra L, et al. Incidence of exercise-induced bronchospasm in Olympic winter sport athletes. Med Sci Sports Exerc 2000;32(4): 732–7.
62. Rundell KW, Spiering BA, Judelson DA, et al. Bronchoconstriction during cross-country skiing: is there really a refractory period? Med Sci Sports Exerc 2003;35: 18–26.
63. Pohjantähti H, Laitinen J, Parkkari J. Exercise-induced bronchospasm among healthy elite cross country skiers and non-athletic students. Scand J Med Sci Sports 2005;15(5):324–8.
64. Sue-Chu M, Brannan JD, Anderson SD, et al. Airway hyperresponsiveness to methacholine, adenosine 5-monophosphate, mannitol, eucapnic voluntary hyperpnoea and field exercise challenge in elite cross-scountry skiers. Br J Sports Med 2010;44(11):827–32.
65. Larsson K, Ohlsén P, Larsson L, et al. High prevalence of asthma in cross country skiers. BMJ 1993;307(6915):1326–9.
66. Stenfors N. Self-reported symptoms and bronchial hyperresponsiveness in elite cross-country skiers. Respir Med 2010;104(11):1760–3.
67. Helenius I, Haahtela T. Allergy and asthma in elite summer sport athletes. J Allergy Clin Immunol 2000;106(3):444–52.
68. Weiler JM, Layton T, Hunt M. Asthma in United States Olympic athletes who participated in the 1996 summer games. J Allergy Clin Immunol 1998;102(5):722–6.
69. Rundell KW, Im J, Mayers LB, et al. Self-reported symptoms and exercise-induced asthma in the elite athlete. Med Sci Sports Exerc 2001;33(2):208–13.
70. Sue-Chu M. Winter sports athletes: long-term effects of cold air exposure. J Sports Med 2012;46(6):397–401.
71. Bernard A, Nickmilder M, Voisin C. Outdoor swimming pools and the risks of asthma and allergies during adolescence. Eur Respir J 2008;32(4):979–88.
72. Bougault V, Boulet LP. Airway dysfunction in swimmers. Br J Sports Med 2012; 46(6):402–6.
73. Helenius I, Rytilä P, Sarna S, et al. Effect of continuing or finishing high-level sports on airway inflammation, bronchial hyperresponsiveness, and asthma: a 5-year prospective follow-up study of 42 highly trained swimmers. J Allergy Clin Immunol 2002;109(6):962–8.
74. Castricum A, Holzer K, Brukner P, et al. The role of the bronchial provocation challenge tests in the diagnosis of exercise-induced bronchoconstriction in elite swimmers. Br J Sports Med 2010;44(10):736–40.
75. Beuther DA, Martin RJ. Efficacy of a heat exchanger mask in cold exercise-induced asthma. Chest 2006;129(5):1188–93.

Where to from Here for Exercise-Induced Bronchoconstriction
The Unanswered Questions

Teal S. Hallstrand, MD, MPH[a],*, Pascale Kippelen, PhD[b],
Johan Larsson, MD[c], Valérie Bougault, PhD[d],
Janneke C. van Leeuwen, MD[e], Jean M.M. Driessen, MD, PhD[f],
John D. Brannan, PhD[g]

KEYWORDS

- Injury • Epithelium • Water transport • Mast cells • Sensory nerves • Eicosanoids

KEY POINTS

- Injury of the epithelium is important in the development of exercise-induced bronchoconstriction (EIB).
- Airway injury in elite athletes may relate to the large volumes of air inspired during training.
- Dysregulation of water movement and balance in the airways may contribute to the pathology of EIB.
- Mast cells, eosinophils, and sensory nerve cells are all likely to be involved in EIB.
- Cysteinyl leukotrienes are the major mediators of EIB with prostaglandins (PGs) likely to play a role in attenuating (PGE_2) or enhancing (PGD_2) the response.
- Refractoriness after exercise may relate to desensitization of airway receptors rather than depletion of mediators.
- New and more sensitive technologies for assaying mediators and measuring changes in pulmonary function are becoming available and will improve our understanding of EIB.

Continued

Conflict of Interest: T.S. Hallstrand has received research grants from the NIH, American Lung Association, has served as a consultant for Amgen and TEVA pharmaceuticals, and has received lecture fees from Merck & Co.
[a] Division of Pulmonary and Critical Care, University of Washington, Department of Medicine, 1959 NE Pacific Street, Box 356166, Seattle, WA 98195-6522, USA; [b] Centre for Sports Medicine & Human Performance, Brunel University, Kingston lane, Uxbridge, Middlesex UB8 3PH, UK; [c] Lung and Allergy Research, Division of Respiratory Medicine and Allergy, Department of Medicine, Karolinska Institutet, Karolinska University Hospital, Huddinge, Stockholm, Sweden; [d] Faculty of Sport sciences, Université Lille Nord de France (Lille 2 University of Health and Law), E.A. 4488, 59790, France; [e] Department of Pediatrics, Medisch Spectrum Twente, Enschede 7513 ER, The Netherlands; [f] Department of Sports Medicine, Tjongerschans Hospital, Heerenveen, The Netherlands; [g] Department of Respiratory & Sleep Medicine, Westmead Hospital, University of Sydney, Westmead, New South Wales 2145, Australia
* Corresponding author.
E-mail address: tealh@uw.edu

Immunol Allergy Clin N Am 33 (2013) 423–442
http://dx.doi.org/10.1016/j.iac.2013.02.010
0889-8561/13/$ – see front matter © 2013 Elsevier Inc. All rights reserved.

immunology.theclinics.com

Continued

- Mild EIB may represent a different phenotype than more severe EIB and involve different mechanisms.
- EIB in children has faster onset and recovery compared with adults and the mechanism for this may relate to remodeling.

WHAT IS THE ROLE OF INJURY OF THE EPITHELIUM IN EXERCISE-INDUCED BRONCHOCONSTRICTION?

In recent years, a concept has emerged placing an abnormal airway epithelium at the center of asthma development and progression.[1,2] In asthmatic patients, properties of the epithelial barrier are believed to be impaired as a result of both intrinsic (eg, genetic polymorphisms)[3] and environmental factors (such as respiratory viruses, cigarette smoke, pollution, and allergens).[4–7] Susceptibility of the epithelium to damage by environmental agents followed by incomplete repair is believed to lead to a dysregulated repair process, with secretion of biologically active substances that drive the structural and inflammatory changes characteristic of asthma.[8] *In vitro* studies have recently confirmed that (1) the bronchial epithelial barrier in asthma is compromised (facilitating penetration of allergens and other noxious airborne particles) and (2) bronchial epithelial cells from asthmatic patients are inherently dysfunctional in their ability to repair wounds.[9,10] Whether these pathologic changes can be observed specifically in the airways of patients with exercise-induced bronchoconstriction (EIB) is not known; however, the number of ciliated epithelial cells shed into the airway lumen is higher in patients with asthma who have EIB.[11]

Although 10% of the population have EIB, this percentage is higher in elite athletes, making it one of the most common morbidities in this group.[12] High minute ventilation in conditions with dry air and a high pollen count may be factors that increase the incidence of EIB.[13–15] There is a connection between the incidence and the number of training years and intensity of the sport[16] suggesting that repetitive injury may play a role. It has been proposed that repetitive epithelial injury and the repair process that follows in elite athletes contributes to the development of EIB, possibly as a result of a change in contractile properties of the bronchial smooth muscle.[17,18]

Previous investigations *in vivo* based on indirect measures of airway epithelial integrity (ie, the concentration of columnar epithelial cells in induced sputum) suggest that injury to the airway epithelium is a key susceptibility factor for asthma with EIB.[19] Animal-based[20,21] and human-based studies[11,22–24] suggest that exercise hyperpnoea can lead to a transient loss of the integrity of the airway epithelial barrier. However, confirmation is required on whether the airway epithelium of patients with EIB (with and without asthma) is structurally and functionally abnormal.

Support for a central role of injury of the airway epithelium in EIB is important in that it may prompt a novel therapeutic approach to treatment. Whereas the currently recognized treatments for EIB (eg, inhaled β_2-agonists and inhaled corticosteroids [ICS]) act mainly downstream from the airway injury (regulating the inflammatory process, mucus secretion, and airway hyperresponsiveness), drugs that help to restore normal epithelial function could potentially prevent the inception of the disease and/or alter its course. New therapeutic agents possibly include drugs such as epidermal and keratinocyte growth factors that enhance the ability of the epithelium to withstand environmental challenge and/or to restore the barrier functions.[25,26]

IS THE AIRWAY SURFACE FLUID VOLUME DYSREGULATED?

During exercise, strict regulation of the airway surface liquid is required for effective mucociliary transport, and for humidifying the inhaled air to prevent dehydration of the distal airways.[27] Mathematical models suggest that, during exercise, the rate of water lost by evaporation can exceed the rate of water return with a net loss of water in some generations of airways.[28,29] Breathing dry air at high flow decreases mucociliary clearance to a greater degree in asthmatic individuals than in healthy people.[27] It is possible that an increase in basement membrane thickness in those with asthma[30] may contribute to a slower rate of return of water to the airway surface but this has not been investigated. Treatment with ICS can reverse the changes in thickness[31] and the same treatment reduces the severity of EIB. Several lines of human-based research suggest that disorders of water transport may be a contributor to EIB. A problem in airway fluid regulation has been proposed to lead to mucus hypersecretion and mucosal edema,[32] and in exacerbation of the dehydration stress to the airways during exercise hyperpnoea.[33,34] It has been proposed that the protective effect of the cromones may play a role in epithelial volume regulation through an action on chloride ion channels.[35]

Davis and colleagues[36] prospectively analyzed the effect of inhaling dry air in a canine model of EIB and found that exposure to dry air leads to an inflammatory response and remodeling in this model. In elite skiers, a similar effect from frequent exposure to dry air occurs and an increase in basement membrane thickness has been reported that is similar to asthmatics.[37] Although almost all athletes developed an increase in the thickness of the basement membrane, almost half of the population did not develop EIB or asthmalike symptoms. The reasons why some individuals respond to dry air exposure in such a way that leads to asthma is not fully understood. The early identification of those who will or who will not develop EIB or airway hyperresponsiveness would enable early intervention to prevent further pathologic conditions.

WHAT IS THE ROLE OF AQUAPORINS?

The airway surface liquid volume is regulated by active ion transport and the passive movement of water through membrane water channels called aquaporins (AQPs).[38] There are some differences among species regarding these channels, but there is evidence that AQPs 3 and 4 are predominantly located on the basolateral surface of ciliated and basal epithelial cells, respectively, whereas AQP5 may be located on the apical membrane. Dynamic regulation of expression of some of the AQP subtypes (particularly AQP5) may be involved in restoring the airway surface volume in response to changes in osmolarity.[39] *In vitro* studies indicate that hypertonic stress induces AQP1 and AQP5 expression,[39,40] therefore it is possible that a dysregulation of AQP expression contributes to EIB and this needs to be investigated.

DOES THE SWIMMING POOL ENVIRONMENT CONTRIBUTE TO AIRWAY INJURY?

The ambient levels of many byproducts resulting from the use of different disinfectants including ozone, chlorine, and bromine are not always measured in pool environments, despite existing recommendations.[41] Uncertainties still exist on the effect of these byproducts on health, either genotoxic, toxicologic, or carcinogenic, when they are repeatedly inhaled or absorbed at various concentrations. Potential genotoxic effects have recently been suggested after regular exposure to chlorinated swimming pools but further studies should determine the relative risk of such exposures.[42]

The relationship between trichloramine (NCl_3) concentrations in the swimming pool environment and upper or lower airway injury need to be confirmed.[43] The mechanism by which exposure to trichloramines can contribute to the development of allergic diseases, rhinitis, and/or airway hyperresponsiveness remain to be investigated. Further studies should focus on the contribution of NCl_3 to oxidative stress, epithelial damage, inflammation, and remodeling. The time course and efficiency of airway epithelial repair after inhalation of chlorine byproducts is also currently unknown in swimmers. Overall, the risks-benefits balance of swimming activities (particularly when repeated and intense) remains to be studied in people attending chlorinated swimming pools. Further study is needed to determine if healthy adult and child swimmers, both recreational and competitive, lifeguard attendants, and those with respiratory disorders are vulnerable to the effects of inhaled chlorinated byproducts.

More studies are needed on the optimal preventative measures and management of upper and lower airway disorders in swimmers and these measures need to be adequately implemented. A recent study showed that in swimmers complaining of rhinitis symptoms, the inflammation was mostly neutrophilic,[44] suggesting that ICS could have limited benefit in this condition. Anticholinergic drugs and/or regular nasal irrigation with a saline solution may be considered. Nutritional interventions, through supplementation with omega 3 or antioxidants, may reduce airway hyperresponsiveness in elite swimmers,[45] reduce mucus accumulation, epithelial hyperplasia, and airway hyperresponsiveness after exposure to chlorine, as shown in a recent animal study,[46] but their effects remain to be better documented in humans.

DOES THE EPITHELIUM REGULATE LEUKOCYTE ACTIVATION?

Although it is possible that the movement of water out of the airways during exercise challenge leads directly to the activation of leukocytes or sensory nerves in the airways, a more unifying concept is that movement of water in the airways initiates events within the epithelium causing activation of airway leukocytes. It is clear that water transport or the addition of an osmolar solution to the airways is sensed by the epithelium, leading to the passive movement of water from the epithelial cells to restore the airway surface liquid osmolarity and volume.[47–49] These events maintain the osmolarity of airway surface liquid, but are also accompanied by cellular signaling events that lead to the release of cellular adenosine triphosphate (ATP) and adenosine, the activation of chloride channels, and an increase in intracellular calcium in the epithelium.[48]

The connection between the epithelial response to water loss and the activation of airway leukocytes needs to be understood in much greater detail. One possibility is that the eicosanoid precursor arachidonic acid or an intermediate in the leukotriene synthetic pathway is released by the epithelium leading to production of eicosanoids that mediate bronchoconstriction via a transcellular metabolism.[50,51] Another possibility is that the epithelium releases an enzyme that increases eicosanoid production in leukocytes.[52] One candidate for this role is secreted phospholipase A_2 group X ($sPLA_2$-X), which is the predominant $sPLA_2$ in the airway epithelium[53]; preliminary evidence indicates that $sPLA_2$-X is released into the airways after exercise challenge in individuals with asthma.[54] The release of $sPLA_2$-X by the epithelium may be important in the pathogenesis of EIB because leukocytes such as eosinophils are activated to release leukotrienes by this epithelial-derived enzyme.[55] As differentiated cultures of primary human airway epithelial cells in organotypic culture are now possible, much more work should be conducted on the epithelial response to water transfer and the nature of the products that are released by epithelial cells in response to this stimulus. The release of specific epithelial-derived products that are identified will need to be examined using *in vivo* model systems of EIB. In this regard, animal models that can capitalize on the revolution in molecular immunology using genetically altered organisms should be further developed. A well-described murine model of EIB has not been developed although there is a well-described canine model of EIB.[56] Other species such as guinea pigs also develop hyperpnea-induced bronchoconstriction even in the absence of sensitization, but genetic alterations in these animals are not readily achieved at this time.

WHAT IS THE CONTRIBUTION OF THE SENSORY NERVES?

Sensory nerves in the airways may serve as a final common pathway leading to bronchoconstriction in EIB, but many of the specific details about this pathway remain unanswered. Early studies using inhaled lidocaine to prevent EIB did not support a role of sensory nerve afferent pathways[57,58]; however, subsequent studies with neurokinin (NK)$_1$ receptor antagonists in human subjects suggested that there might be some efficacy in blocking this pathway.[59,60] When activated, C-fibers from sensory nerves initiate the release of tachykinins via retrograde axonal transmission.[61,62] C-fibers transmit this activation signal to goblet cells and airway smooth muscle, leading to goblet cell degranulation and mucus release.[32,63] Sensory nerves are activated by eicosanoids, and the activation threshold for sensory nerves is decreased in the presence of leukotrienes.[64,65] Other eicosanoids such as prostaglandin (PG)D$_2$ that cause bronchoconstriction in humans could also act via sensory nerves, although PGD$_2$ can also have direct effects on airway smooth muscle via thromboxane receptors.[66] A major limitation to understanding this system in humans is that the predominant tachykinin in humans is NK A, which has high affinity for the NK$_2$ receptor; substance P is present in humans at lower levels and predominantly binds to the NK$_1$ receptor.[67,68] As receptor antagonists become available for the 3 different NK receptors (ie, NK$_1$, NK$_2$, NK$_3$), a better understanding of the role of sensory nerves in EIB can be ascertained. The sensory nerve system may act as a target for eicosanoids in the airways and may initiate the activation of leukocytes that are in close proximity to airway nerves.

Sensory nerves are also stimulated by changes in osmolarity[69] and coughing is a common feature of hyperpnea with dry air and inhalation of hyperosmolar and hyposmolar aerosols.[70,71] In studies of nasal challenge with hyperosmolar stimuli, there was a significant increase in 15-hydroxyeicosatetranoic acid (15-HETE) in allergic but not healthy individuals.[72] 15-HETE is derived from the epithelium[73] and is an endogenous ligand for the vanilloid receptor TRPV$_1$.

IS MAST CELL INFILTRATION OF THE EPITHELIUM IMPORTANT IN EIB?

Mast cells have long been postulated to play a central role in the pathogenesis of EIB, in part as a result of the effectiveness of cromones to prevent EIB and the responses to surrogates of exercise.[35,74,75] Mast cell degranulation after exercise challenge has been specifically demonstrated in individuals with EIB.[19] These findings have led to the presumption that mast cell infiltration of the airways may be a defining susceptibility feature of patients with EIB. Little work has been done, however, to characterize differences in mast cell populations in the airways or the potential regulation of such mast cell populations. A recent study identified an increase in the expression of tryptase and carboxypeptidase A3 (CPA3) genes in the airway epithelium in asthma, particularly in the Th2 high molecular phenotype of asthma[76]; further study found that the number of intraepithelial mast cells was increased in the Th2 high phenotype of asthma (**Fig. 1**).[77] As the development of mast cell granules and possibly mast cell

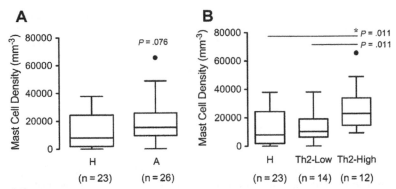

Fig. 1. Density of mast cells, within airway epithelium, among subjects stratified by disease status (*A*) and by Th2 subgroup (*B*). Lines represent median values and boxes represent interquartile ranges. A, asthmatic; H, healthy. *P = .011, Kruskal-Wallis test. (*Reproduced from* Dougherty RH, Sidhu SS, Raman K, et al. Accumulation of intraepithelial mast cells with a unique protease phenotype in T(H)2-high asthma. J Allergy Clin Immunol 2010;125:1046–53; with permission.)

function can be regulated in peripheral tissues, these findings are particularly notable as mucosal mast cells typically do not express CPA3.[78] A study comparing airway cell gene expression obtained by induced sputum found that both tryptase and CPA3 genes were among the most differentially overexpressed in asthmatics with EIB relative to asthmatics without EIB, especially after exercise challenge.[79] More studies are needed in this area to delineate the mast cell population in the airway epithelium and airway wall of patients with EIB, and the regulation of such mast cell populations by the airway epithelium.

WHAT IS THE ROLE OF LIPID MEDIATORS?

Several lines of evidence demonstrate the overproduction of certain inflammatory eicosanoids such as the cysteinyl leukotrienes (CysLTs) and PGD_2 in patients with EIB. Mast cells are the major source of PGD_2. A significant increase in the urinary excretion of 11β-$PGF_{2\alpha}$, a metabolite of PGD_2, has been observed after exercise,[80] eucapnic voluntary hyperpnea with dry air,[81,82] and inhaled mannitol, which serves as a surrogate for exercise challenge.[75] An important unanswered question is whether PGD_2 plays a causal role in the development of EIB. The increase in PGD_2 is related to the % decrease in forced expiratory volume in the first second of expiration (FEV_1) after eucapnic voluntary hyperpnea (**Fig. 2**).[81] Further drugs that attenuate EIB, including sodium cromoglycate[75,81] and beclomethasone,[82] prevent the increase in PGD_2 after challenge (**Fig. 3**).[81–83] In response to mannitol, there is a relationship between the change in urinary levels of 11β-$PGF_{2\alpha}$ and the change in leukotriene $(LT)E_4$,[84] suggesting that LTE_4 is also likely to be released from mast cells or that the release occurs in parallel (**Fig. 4**). Whether this same relationship occurs in response to exercise in those with or without sputum eosinophilia is not known. Eosinophils are a potential source of CysLTs. Studies have also reported an increase in the urinary concentration of both 11β-$PGF_{2\alpha}$ and LTE_4 after challenge with mannitol and exercise in nonasthmatics without airway hyperresponsivenss.[85–87]

Lipid mediators such as CysLTs and PGD_2 are eicosanoids that are derived from arachidonic acid.[88] There are also protective lipid mediators that are derived from

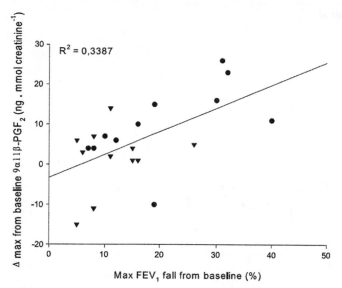

Fig. 2. Correlation between the degree of bronchoconstriction after eucapnic voluntary hyperpnea and excretion of urinary 9α11β-PGF$_2$ in athletes with EIB after administration of placebo (*circles*) or 40 mg of sodium cromoglycate (*triangles*). (*Reproduced from* Kippelen P, Larsson J, Anderson SD, et al. Effect of sodium cromoglycate on mast cell mediators during hyperpnea in athletes. Med Sci Sports Exerc 2010;42:1853–60; with permission.)

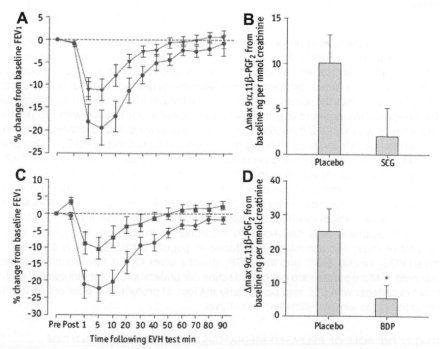

Fig. 3. (*A, C*) The percentage change in FEV$_1$ from baseline and (*B, D*) maximum change in 9α11β-PGF$_2$ in response to 6 minutes of eucapnic voluntary hyperpnea (EVH) with dry air (*A, B*) in the presence of placebo (*closed circles*) and after sodium cromoglycate (*inverted triangles*) in 11 subjects with greater than 10% decrease in FEV$_1$ and (*C, D*) 4.5 hours after placebo (*closed circles*) and 1500 μg of beclomethasone (*squares*) in 8 subjects with asthma. (*Reproduced from* Anderson SD, Kippelen P. Stimulus and mechanism of exercise-induced bronchoconstriction. Breathe 2010;7:25–33; with permission.)

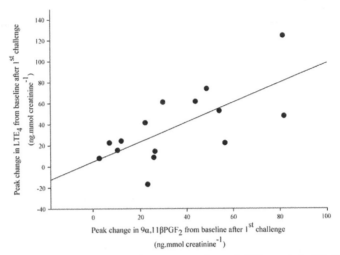

Fig. 4. Correlation between the peak concentration of LTE_4 and $9\alpha11\beta$-PGF_2 after a mannitol challenge. r = 0.686, P<.005, n = 15. (*Reproduced from* Larsson J, Perry CP, Anderson SD, et al. The occurrence of refractoriness and mast cell mediator release following mannitol-induced bronchoconstriction. J Appl Physiol 2011;110:1029–35; with permission.)

the same arachidonic acid precursor and a range of other protective mediators that are derived from the metabolism of related free fatty acids other than arachidonic acid.[89] The regulation of eicosanoid formation is complex, can involve transcellular metabolism, and is often dictated by the terminal synthetic enzyme within a cell. One study found that the levels of the protective lipid mediator lipoxin A_4 decreased after exercise challenge and that the levels were lower in asthmatics with EIB relative to asthmatics without EIB.[90] Another mediator in the airways that decreases after exercise challenge in individuals with EIB but not normal individuals is PGE_2.[11] One possibility is that the reduction in the production of these mediators (ie, PGE_2 and LXA_4) represents epithelial dysfunction in asthma. Epithelial cells treated with interleukin (IL)-13 *in vitro* have reduced capacity for PGE_2 synthesis through a reduction in the synthetic enzymes cyclooxygenase-2 (COX-2) and PGE synthase 1.[91] Epithelial cells normally have an inhibitory effect on mast cell activation, but this protective effect is reduced in epithelial cells derived from individuals with asthma, suggesting that a regulator of mast cell activation is reduced in people with EIB.[92] It is known that inhaled PGE_2 inhibits EIB[93] and that PGE_2 directly alters CysLT formation in cultured mast cells.[94] More studies are needed to refine our understanding of eicosanoid metabolism in patients with EIB, and particularly the loss of protective mediators related to alterations in the airway epithelium in asthma.

WHAT IS THE ROLE OF RELEASED MEDIATORS AND THE DEVELOPMENT OF REFRACTORINESS?

Refractoriness is defined as a decrease in the airway response to repeated challenge with the same stimulus within 2 to 4 hours of the initial stimulus. A decrease in release of mediators of bronchoconstriction on repeated challenge was proposed as a possible mechanism,[95] but subsequent studies have not supported this hypothesis.[84,96] Because of the inhibitory effect of indomethacin on refractoriness, PGE_2 has been suggested to play a vital role[97–101] although no studies have confirmed this directly.

Conflicting results have been documented when the first challenge is performed breathing hot humid air and the second challenge breathing dry air, and this needs further investigation. Three studies found protection from dry air challenge after an initial exercise challenge while inhaling hot humid air.[102–104] This protection was abolished by indomethacin. In complete contrast, 2 other investigators reported severe EIB after breathing dry room air 20 minutes after an initial exercise breathing hot humid air **(Fig. 5)**.[105,106]

Although the occurrence of refractoriness after repeated challenge with exercise or surrogates of exercise may be dependent on mediator release, the occurrence of a protective effect after exercise challenge with humid air, in the absence of EIB, seems at odds with other results. Research is needed to investigate possible common links between the challenges; adenosine is one possible link. The change in airway surface liquid volume that may be expected to occur during challenge by exercise, eucapnic voluntary hyperpnea, distilled water, hypertonic saline, and mannitol is likely to lead to ATP release.[48] The ATP released can then be converted to adenosine and exert effects via the A_{2b} receptor to maintain the airway surface liquid volume.[48] The A_{2b} receptor is also the receptor on mast cells that causes mediator release when stimulated by adenosine.[107] Adenosine has been measured in expired breath condensate during EIB and there was a significant relationship between the increase in concentration of adenosine and the percent decrease in FEV_1.[108]

Many of the early studies in the 1980s and early 1990s focused on the pulmonary response with little interest in the molecular mechanisms underlying the refractory period. It is now well established that the release of mediators is involved in EIB,

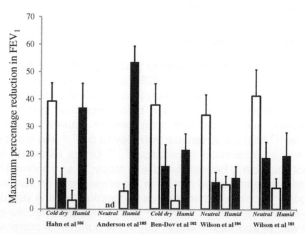

Fig. 5. Maximum percentage decrease in FEV_1 (mean ± SD) after exercise compared with values before exercise. The first challenge (*open bars*) was performed breathing either dry air (cold or room temperature) or humid air; the second challenge (*closed bars*) was always performed breathing dry air. Refractoriness was seen in all studies when the first challenge was performed breathing dry air but not with humid air. In the studies by Hahn and colleagues[106] and Anderson and colleagues,[105] no protective effect was seen during the second challenge when hot humid air was inspired during the first challenge. However, in the other studies by Ben Dov and colleagues[102] and by Wilson and colleagues,[103,104] a protective effect was seen during the second challenge when the first challenge was performed breathing humid air. The values are reproduced from the original data given.

and the technology available to measure biological pathways has improved. There is now greater availability of specific inhibitors of mediator synthesis as well as specific agonists and antagonists of the respective receptors for each mediator. These agents may reveal the specific mediators, in addition to CysLTs, that contribute to broncho-constriction in EIB. For example, the evidence for the involvement of PGs is based on the effect of non-specific COX inhibitors, which indicates a role for PGE_2; however, no further conclusion can be drawn. When studying the effects of different drugs not only the pulmonary response but also mediator release needs to be taken into consideration. Similarly some PGD_2 antagonists have been shown to provide no benefit against EIB.[109] More specific antagonists to a wider range of receptors for PGD_2 and its metabolites may become available and need to be tested.

Another great advantage is the development of increasingly sensitive and specific methods for measuring the various mediators. The possibility of performing metabolomics will be a great help in the search for new mediators and in understanding the relationship between the currently known mediators. Until now, much of our knowledge on the mechanism of EIB was based on the levels of LTE_4 and the PGD_2 metabolite 11β-$PGF_{2\alpha}$.[80–82,110] Using lipidomics, it will be possible to study several mediators and their metabolites simultaneously in the same sample, and compare patterns of release and their dynamics. The ability to measure mediators in different media (eg, sputum, saliva, urine, blood) before, during, and after challenge will also help to increase our understanding of the mechanism of EIB.

Additional studies are needed to investigate the reproducibility of the refractory period. It will be important to understand if variability in the refractory period among individuals is related to airway smooth muscle sensitivity, revealing a phenotype of the airway smooth muscle or other factors such as the intensity of cellular inflammation. A recent proposal that remains to be proved is that the high levels of CysLTs lead to desensitization of the CysLT receptor.[84]

IS MILD EIB A DIFFERENT PHENOTYPE?

There are several observations that suggest that mild EIB may be a different phenotype than moderate or severe EIB. Mild EIB can be considered as less than 15% decrease in FEV_1 after exercise and possibly less than 20% decrease in FEV_1 in those with a normal percentage predicted value before exercise. Mild EIB is commonly observed in athletes and people with symptoms of asthma but without a formal asthma diagnosis.[111] Mild EIB is variable from day to day[112] and may benefit from dietary[86,113–116] and environmental influences.[117,118] Unlike moderate to severe EIB, mild EIB may not necessarily be associated with atopy,[111] an abnormal fractional concentration of nitric oxide in expired gas,[119] or the presence of sputum eosinophilia.[120] Mild EIB may occur in cold-weather athletes suggesting that the vasculature may be contributing to airway narrowing.[121] Inhaled β_2 agonists are effective in mild EIB but daily treatment with β_2 agonists results in loss in the duration of protection, slower recovery from EIB, and sometimes an increase in the severity of EIB.[122–125] Daily treatment with ICS is effective against mild to severe EIB although low doses of ICS may not be as effective as high doses of ICS.[126] Drugs such as sodium cromoglycate or nedocromil sodium[74] and montelukast acutely inhibit mild to severe EIB[127] but not everyone is protected to the same extent. One important question is whether to treat mild EIB without symptoms, or treat mild EIB with symptoms with an inhaled β_2 agonist alone when required. It will also be important to understand the factors that lead to the progression of EIB severity in some individuals and if this can be prevented by early treatment.

WHAT IS THE BENEFIT OF LONG-TERM ICS ON EIB IN PERSONS WITH ASTHMA?

Few studies have investigated the treatment of EIB using regular ICS beyond a period of 12 weeks[128]; many studies have focused on the benefits soon after introducing an ICS.[126] If the airway response to exercise and other indirect tests demonstrates a link between airway inflammation and a sensitive airway smooth muscle as previously proposed,[129] then resolution of EIB after ICS suggests the link between these 2 key features of asthma has been abolished with treatment. It is likely that both eosinophils and mast cells are sensitive to corticosteroid treatment and that mast cells may take longer to respond to treatment than eosinophils. An important question is whether the resolution of EIB in a person with asthma is a reliable objective marker of clinical control. Similarly, it will be important to examine the benefit of ICS in athletes who have EIB and asthma, and those who have EIB alone.

IS THERE A ROLE FOR THE ANTICHOLINERGIC DRUGS?

There is evidence to suggest that vagal tone of the airway smooth muscle may play an important role in the susceptibility to EIB. The variable efficacy of anticholinergic drugs in EIB may be due to variations in cardiac vagal activity that have implied that vagal stimulation may be important.[130,131] There are an increasing number of anticholinergic drugs that may help resolve this question and determine if this variability in response is due to the potency of the drug. To date, few studies, if any, have investigated the use of these stronger anticholinergic drugs on EIB.

WHY DO CHILDREN GET EIB MORE QUICKLY AND RECOVER MORE QUICKLY?

It has been shown that many asthmatic children with EIB can have breakthrough EIB (ie, the onset of bronchoconstriction *during* exercise) within minutes after the start of exercise.[132,133] Breakthrough EIB is accompanied by a more severe decrease in pulmonary function after exercise, and therefore apparently a sign of uncontrolled asthma.[133] Moreover, breakthrough EIB is a frustrating symptom that may result in premature withdrawal of a child from play and sports. We need to know which medications are best for prevention of the phenomenon of breakthrough EIB. A suggested mechanism to account for breakthrough EIB is an imbalance between bronchoconstrictor mediators (probably mast cell in origin) and bronchodilator PGs (probably epithelial in origin). The early breakthrough EIB observed in children compared with adults may be caused by differences in the proximity of the mast cells to the airway surface and their density, and the ability of the epithelium to produce PGE_2. In children, there is a shorter time to maximal bronchoconstriction and quicker recovery from EIB than has been described in adults.[134–136] The time course of bronchoconstriction after exercise is age related and the younger the child, the shorter the time to maximal bronchoconstriction after exercise (**Fig. 6**).[134] The mechanism responsible for this difference between children and adults is unknown but may relate to differences in the epithelium or the site of mast cells. For example, a faster change in osmolarity may occur in children compared with adults, which may result in a more rapid onset of mediator release. It is unknown whether this cascade indeed happens faster at younger age.

The quick onset and recovery of EIB in young children could also be the result of a shortened response and relaxation time of the airway smooth muscle in airways of younger children. The age-related response of airway smooth muscle may partially be due to airway remodeling and a change in airway geometry with older age. Deep inspirations, as happen at the start of exercise, usually have a

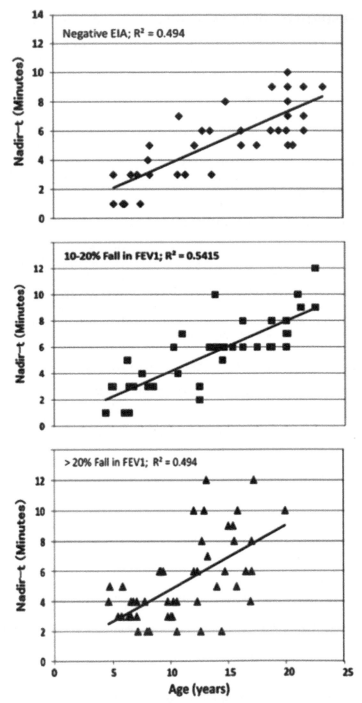

Fig. 6. The correlation between age and time to Nadir (Nadir-t). Data are divided according to potential cutoffs or a negative test. Each sign represents a single participant. (*Reproduced from* Vilozni D, Szeinberg A, Barak A, et al. The relation between age and time to maximal bronchoconstriction following exercise in children. Respir Med 2009;103:1456–60; with permission.)

bronchodilating effect in asthmatic children and healthy adults,[137] which is believed to be caused by relaxation of the airway smooth muscle.[138] This potent bronchodilating mechanism may fail in remodeled airways of adult asthmatics, as if the airway smooth muscle has become frozen and fails to fluidize.[138] Remodeling of the airways in asthmatic adults may hinder stretch-induced relaxation of smooth muscle find prevent the rapid onset of bronchoconstriction caused by stiffening of the airway smooth muscle cytoskeleton.[138] There is a lack of longitudinal studies on the evolution of EIB and breakthrough EIB from young asthmatic children into adulthood.

REFERENCES

1. Holgate ST. Epithelium dysfunction in asthma. J Allergy Clin Immunol 2007;120: 1233–44.
2. Swindle EJ, Collins JE, Davies DE. Breakdown in epithelial barrier function in patients with asthma: identification of novel therapeutic approaches. J Allergy Clin Immunol 2009;124:23–34 [quiz: 35–6].
3. Moffatt MF, Gut IG, Demenais F, et al. A large-scale, consortium-based genome-wide association study of asthma. N Engl J Med 2010;363:1211–21.
4. Jacquet A. Interactions of airway epithelium with protease allergens in the allergic response. Clin Exp Allergy 2011;41:305–11.
5. Wark PA, Johnston SL, Bucchieri F, et al. Asthmatic bronchial epithelial cells have a deficient innate immune response to infection with rhinovirus. J Exp Med 2005;201:937–47.
6. Hackett TL, Singhera GK, Shaheen F, et al. Intrinsic phenotypic differences of asthmatic epithelium and its inflammatory responses to respiratory syncytial virus and air pollution. Am J Respir Cell Mol Biol 2011;45:1090–100.
7. Xiao C, Puddicombe SM, Field S, et al. Defective epithelial barrier function in asthma. J Allergy Clin Immunol 2011;128:549–56.
8. Davies DE, Holgate ST. Asthma: the importance of epithelial mesenchymal communication in pathogenesis. Inflammation and the airway epithelium in asthma. Int J Biochem Cell Biol 2002;34:1520–6.
9. Stevens PT, Kicic A, Sutanto EN, et al. Dysregulated repair in asthmatic paediatric airway epithelial cells: the role of plasminogen activator inhibitor-1. Clin Exp Allergy 2008;38:1901–10.
10. Kicic A, Hallstrand TS, Sutanto EN, et al. Decreased fibronectin production significantly contributes to dysregulated repair of asthmatic epithelium. Am J Respir Crit Care Med 2010;181:889–98.
11. Hallstrand TS, Moody MW, Wurfel MM, et al. Inflammatory basis of exercise-induced bronchoconstriction. Am J Respir Crit Care Med 2005;172:679–86.
12. Fitch KD. An overview of asthma and airwayhyperresponsiveness in Olympic athletes. Br J Sports Med 2012;46:413–6.
13. Helenius I, Rytilä P, Sarna S, et al. Effect of continuing or finishing high-level sports on airway inflammation, bronchial hyperresponsiveness, and asthma: a 5-year prospective follow-up study of 42 highly trained swimmers. J Allergy Clin Immunol 2002;109:962–8.
14. Leuppi JD, Kuln M, Comminot C, et al. High prevalence of bronchial hyperresponsiveness and asthma in ice hockey players. Eur Respir J 1998;12:13–6.
15. Karjalainen J, Lindqvist A, Laitenen LA. Seasonal variability of exercise-induced asthma especially out-doors. Effect of birch pollen allergy. Clin Exp Allergy 1989;19:273–9.

16. Knoepfli BH, Luke-Zeitoun M, von Duvillard SP, et al. A high incidence of exercise-induced bronchoconstriction in triathletes of the Swiss National Team. Br J Sports Med 2007;41:486–91.

17. Anderson SD, Kippelen P. Exercise-induced bronchoconstriction: pathogenesis. Curr Allergy Asthma Rep 2005;5:116–22.

18. Anderson SD, Kippelen P. Airway injury as a mechanism for exercise-induced bronchoconstriction in elite athletes. J Allergy Clin Immunol 2008;122:225–35.

19. Hallstrand TS, Moody MW, Aitken ML, et al. Airway immunopathology of asthma with exercise-induced bronchoconstriction. J Allergy Clin Immunol 2005;116:586–93.

20. Omori C, Schofield BH, Mitzner W, et al. Hyperpnea with dry air causes time-dependent alterations in mucosal morphology and bronchovascular permeability. J Appl Physiol 1995;78:1043–51.

21. Barbet JP, Chauveau N, Labbe S, et al. Breathing dry air causes acute epithelial damage and inflammation of the guinea pig trachea. J Appl Physiol 1988;64:1851–7.

22. Bolger C, Tufvesson E, Sue-Chu M, et al. Hyperpnea-induced bronchoconstriction and urinary CC16 levels in athletes. Med Sci Sports Exerc 2011;43:1207–13.

23. Bolger C, Tufvesson E, Anderson SD, et al. Effect of inspired air conditions on exercise-induced bronchoconstriction and urinary CC16 levels in athletes. J Appl Physiol 2011;111:1059–65.

24. Chimenti L, Morici G, Paternò A, et al. Bronchial epithelial damage after a half-marathon in nonasthmatic amateur runners. Am J Physiol Lung Cell Mol Physiol 2010;298:L857–62.

25. Tillie-Leblond I, Gosset P, Le Berre R, et al. Keratinocyte growth factor improves alterations of lung permeability and bronchial epithelium in allergic rats. Eur Respir J 2007;30:31–9.

26. Basuroy S, Seth A, Elias B, et al. MAPK interacts with occludin and mediates EGF-induced prevention of tight junction disruption by hydrogen peroxide. Biochem J 2006;393:69–77.

27. Daviskas E, Anderson SD, Gonda I, et al. Changes in mucociliary clearance during and after isocapnic hyperventilation in asthmatic and healthy subjects. Eur Respir J 1995;8:742–51.

28. Daviskas E, Gonda I, Anderson SD. Mathematical modelling of the heat and water transport in the human respiratory tract. J Appl Physiol 1990;69:362–72.

29. Daviskas E, Gonda I, Anderson SD. Local airway heat and water vapour losses. Respir Physiol 1991;84:115–32.

30. Ward C, Pais M, Bish R, et al. Airway inflammation, basement membrane thickening and bronchial hyperresponsiveness in asthma. Thorax 2002;57:309–16.

31. Ward C, Walters H. Airway wall remodelling: the influence of corticosteroids. Curr Opin Allergy Clin Immunol 2005;5:43–8.

32. Hallstrand TS, Debley JS, Farin FM, et al. Role of MUC5AC in the pathogenesis of exercise-induced bronchoconstriction. J Allergy Clin Immunol 2007;119:1092–8.

33. Loughlin CE, Esther CRJ, Lazarowski ER, et al. Neutrophilic inflammation is associated with altered airway hydration in stable asthmatics. Respir Med 2010;104:29–33.

34. Park C, Stafford C, Lockette W. Exercise-induced asthma may be associated with diminished sweat secretion rates in humans. Chest 2008;134:552–8.

35. Anderson SD, Rodwell LT, Daviskas E, et al. The protective effect of nedocromil sodium and other drugs on airway narrowing provoked by hyperosmolar stimuli: a role for the airway epithelium. J Allergy Clin Immunol 1996;98:S124–34.

36. Davis MS, Schofield B, Freed AN. Repeated peripheral airway hyperpnea causes inflammation and remodeling in dogs. Med Sci Sports Exerc 2003;35: 608–16.
37. Karjalainen EM, Laitinen A, Sue-Chu M, et al. Evidence of airway inflammation and remodeling in ski athletes with and without bronchial hyperresponsiveness to methacholine. Am J Respir Crit Care Med 2000;161:2086–91.
38. King LS, Yasui M. Aquaporins and disease: lessons from mice and humans. Trends Endocrinol Metab 2002;13:355–60.
39. Hoffert JD, Leitch V, Agre P, et al. Hypertonic induction of aquaporin-5 expression through an ERK-dependent pathway. J Biol Chem 2000;275:9070–7.
40. Leitch V, Agre P, King LS. Altered ubiquination and stability of aquaporin-1 in hypertonic stress. Proc Natl Acad Sci U S A 2001;98:2894–8.
41. World Health Organization. International programme on chemical safety, environmental health criteria 216: disinfectants and disinfectant by-products. Geneva (Switzerland): WHO; 2000.
42. Kogevinas M, Villanueva CM, Font-Ribera L, et al. Genotoxic effects in swimmers exposed to disinfection by-products in indoor swimming pools. Environ Health Perspect 2010;118:1531–7.
43. Fornander L, Ghafouri B, Lindahl M, et al. Airway irritation among indoor swimming pool personnel: trichloramine exposure, exhaled NO and protein profiling of nasal lavage fluids. Int Arch Occup Environ Health 2012. [Epub ahead of print].
44. Gelardi M, Ventura MT, Fiorella R, et al. Allergic and non-allergic rhinitis in swimmers: clinical and cytological aspects. Br J Sports Med 2012;46:54–8.
45. Mickleborough TD. A nutritional approach to managing exercise-induced asthma. Exerc Sport Sci Rev 2008;36:135–44.
46. Fanucchi MV, Bracher A, Doran SF, et al. Post-exposure antioxidant treatment in rats decreases airway hyperplasia and hyperreactivity due to chlorine inhalation. Am J Respir Cell Mol Biol 2012;46:599–606.
47. Matsui H, Davis CW, Tarran R, et al. Osmotic water permeabilities of cultured, well-differentiated normal and cystic fibrosis airway epithelia. J Clin Invest 2000;105:1419–27.
48. Tarran R. Regulation of airway surface liquid volume and mucus transport by active ion transport. Proc Am Thorac Soc 2004;1:42–6.
49. Willumsen JN, Davis CW, Boucher RC. Selective response of human airway epithelia to luminal but not serosol solution hypertonicity. Possible role for proximal airway epithelia as an osmolality transducer. J Clin Invest 1994;94: 779–87.
50. Peters-Golden M, Feyssa A. Transcellular eicosanoid synthesis in cocultures of alveolar epithelial cells and macrophages. Am J Physiol 1993;264:L438–47.
51. Zarini S, Gijon MA, Ransome AE, et al. Transcellular biosynthesis of cysteinyl leukotrienes in vivo during mouse peritoneal inflammation. Proc Natl Acad Sci U S A 2009;106:8296–301.
52. Holgate ST, Peters-Golden M, Panettieri RA, et al. Roles of cysteinyl leukotrienes in airway inflammation, smooth muscle function, and remodeling. J Allergy Clin Immunol 2003;111:S18–34 [discussion: S34–6].
53. Hallstrand TS, Lai Y, Ni Z, et al. Relationship between levels of secreted phospholipase A groups IIA and X in the airways and asthma severity. Clin Exp Allergy 2011;41:801–10.
54. Hallstrand TS, Chi EY, Singer AG, et al. Secreted phospholipase A2 group X overexpression in asthma and bronchial hyperresponsiveness. Am J Respir Crit Care Med 2007;176:1072–8.

55. Lai Y, Oslund RC, Bollinger JG, et al. Eosinophil cysteinyl leukotriene synthesis mediated by exogenous secreted phospholipase A group X. J Biol Chem 2010; 285:41491–500.

56. Freed AN, Anderson SD. Exercise-induced bronchoconstriction. Animal models. In: Kay AB, Kaplan AP, Bousquet J, et al, editors. Allergy and allergic diseases. Oxford (United Kingdom): Blackwell Scientific Publications; 2008. p. 792–805.

57. Enright PL, McNally JF, Souhrada JF. Effect of lidocaine on the ventilatory and airway responses to exercise in asthmatics. Am Rev Respir Dis 1980;122:823–8.

58. Griffin MP, McFadden ER Jr, Ingram RH Jr, et al. Controlled-analysis of the effects of inhaled lignocaine in exercise-induced asthma. Thorax 1982;37: 741–5.

59. Fahy JV, Wong HH, Geppetti P, et al. Effect of an NK1 receptor antagonist (CP-99,994) on hypertonic saline-induced bronchoconstriction and cough in male asthmatic subjects. Am J Respir Crit Care Med 1995;152:879–84.

60. Ichinose M, Miura M, Yamauchi H, et al. A neurokinin 1-receptor antagonist improves exercise-induced airway narrowing in asthmatic patients. Am J Respir Crit Care Med 1996;153:936–41.

61. Bloomquist EI, Kream RM. Leukotriene D acts in part to contract guinea pig ileum smooth muscle by releasing substance P. J Pharmacol Exp Ther 1987; 240:523–8.

62. Ishikawa J, Ichinose M, Miura M, et al. Involvement of endogenous tachykinins in LTD4-induced airway responses. Eur Respir J 1996;9:486–92.

63. Kuo HP, Rohde JA, Tokuyama K, et al. Capsaicin and sensory neuropeptide stimulation of goblet cell secretion in guinea-pig trachea. J Physiol 1990;431: 629–41.

64. Ellis JL, Undem BJ. Role of peptidoleukotrienes in capsaicin-sensitive sensory fibre-mediated responses in guinea-pig airways. J Physiol 1991;436:469–84.

65. Hwang SW, Cho H, Kwak J, et al. Direct activation of capsaicin receptors by products of lipoxygenases: endogenous capsaicin-like substances. Proc Natl Acad Sci U S A 2000;97:6155–60.

66. Coleman RA, Sheldrick RL. Prostanoid-induced contraction of human bronchial smooth muscle is mediated by TP-receptors. Br J Pharmacol 1989;96:688–92.

67. Barnes PJ. Neurogenic inflammation in the airways. Respir Physiol 2001;125: 145–54.

68. Naline E, Devillier P, Drapeau G, et al. Characterization of neurokinin effects and receptor selectivity in human isolated bronchi. Am Rev Respir Dis 1989;140: 679–86.

69. Pisarri TE, Jonson A, Coleridge HM, et al. Intravenous injection of hypertonic NaCl solutions stimulates pulmonary C-fibres in dogs. Am J Physiol 1991; 260(5 Pt 2):H1522–30.

70. Brannan JD, Anderson SD, Perry CP, et al. The safety and efficacy of inhaled dry powder mannitol as a bronchial provocation test for airway hyperresponsiveness: a phase 3 comparison study with hypertonic (4.5%) saline. Respir Res 2005;6:144.

71. Eschenbacher WL, Boushey HA, Sheppard D. Alteration in osmolarity of inhaled aerosols cause bronchoconstriction and cough, but absence of a permeant anion causes cough alone. Am Rev Respir Dis 1984;129:211–5.

72. Koskela H, Di Sciascio MB, Anderson SD, et al. Nasal hyperosmolar challenge with a dry powder of mannitol in patients with allergic rhinitis. Evidence for epithelial cell involvement. Clin Exp Allergy 2000;30:1627–36.

73. Kumlin M, Hamberg M, Granstrom E, et al. 15(S)-Hydroxyeicosatetraenoic acid is the major arachidonic acid metabolite in human bronchi: association with airway epithelium. Arch Biochem Biophys 1990;282:254–62.

74. Spooner C, Spooner G, Rowe B. Mast-cell stabilising agents to prevent exercise-induced bronchoconstriction. Cochrane Database Syst Rev 2003;(4):CD002307.

75. Brannan JD, Gulliksson M, Anderson SD, et al. Inhibition of mast cell PGD release protects against mannitol-induced airway narrowing. Eur Respir J 2006;27:944–50.

76. Woodruff PG, Boushey HA, Dolganov GM, et al. Genome-wide profiling identifies epithelial cell genes associated with asthma and with treatment response to corticosteroids. Proc Natl Acad Sci U S A 2007;104:15858–63.

77. Dougherty RH, Sidhu SS, Raman K, et al. Accumulation of intraepithelial mast cells with a unique protease phenotype in T(H)2-high asthma. J Allergy Clin Immunol 2010;125:1046–53.

78. Gurish MF, Austen KF. Developmental origin and functional specialization of mast cell subsets. Immunity 2012;37:25–33.

79. Hallstrand TS, Wurfel MM, Lai Y, et al. Transglutaminase 2, a novel regulator of eicosanoid production in asthma revealed by genome-wide expression profiling of distinct asthma phenotypes. PLoS One 2010;5:e8583.

80. O'Sullivan S, Roquet A, Dahlen B, et al. Evidence for mast cell activation during exercise-induced bronchoconstriction. Eur Respir J 1998;12:345–50.

81. Kippelen P, Larsson J, Anderson SD, et al. Effect of sodium cromoglycate on mast cell mediators during hyperpnea in athletes. Med Sci Sports Exerc 2010;42:1853–60.

82. Kippelen P, Larsson J, Anderson SD, et al. Acute effects of beclomethasone on hyperpnea-induced bronchoconstriction. Med Sci Sports Exerc 2010;42:273–80.

83. Anderson SD, Kippelen P. Stimulus and mechanism of exercise-induced bronchoconstriction. Breathe 2010;7:25–33.

84. Larsson J, Perry CP, Anderson SD, et al. The occurrence of refractoriness and mast cell mediator release following mannitol-induced bronchoconstriction. J Appl Physiol 2011;110:1029–35.

85. Brannan JD, Gulliksson M, Anderson SD, et al. Evidence of mast cell activation and leukotriene release after mannitol inhalation. Eur Respir J 2003;22:491–6.

86. Mickleborough TD, Murray RL, Ionescu AA, et al. Fish oil supplementation reduces severity of exercise-induced bronchoconstriction in elite athletes. Am J Respir Crit Care Med 2003;168:1181–9.

87. Caillaud C, Le Creff C, Legros P, et al. Strenuous exercise increases plasmatic and urinary leukotriene E4 in cyclists. Can J Appl Physiol 2003;28:793–806.

88. Hallstrand TS, Henderson WR. Role of leukotrienes in exercise-induced bronchoconstriction. Curr Allergy Asthma Rep 2009;9:18–25.

89. Haworth O, Levy BD. Endogenous lipid mediators in the resolution of airway inflammation. Eur Respir J 2007;30:980–92.

90. Tahan F, Saraymen R, Gumus H. The role of lipoxin A4 in exercise-induced bronchoconstriction in asthma. J Asthma 2008;45:161–4.

91. Trudeau J, Hu H, Chibana K, et al. Selective downregulation of prostaglandin E2-related pathways by the Th2 cytokine IL-13. J Allergy Clin Immunol 2006;117:1446–54.

92. Martin N, Ruddick A, Arthur GK, et al. Primary human airway epithelial cell-dependent inhibition of human lung mast cell degranulation. PLoS One 2012;7:e43545.

93. Melillo E, Woolley KL, Manning PJ, et al. Effect of inhaled PGE on exercise-induced bronchoconstriction in asthmatic subjects. Am J Respir Crit Care Med 1994;149:1138–41.

94. Feng C, Beller EM, Bagga S, et al. Human mast cells express multiple EP receptors for prostaglandin E that differentially modulate activation responses. Blood 2006;107:3243–50.

95. Edmunds A, Tooley M, Godfrey S. The refractory period after exercise-induced asthma: its duration and relation to the severity of exercise. Am Rev Respir Dis 1978;117:247–54.

96. Belcher NG, Murdoch R, Dalton N, et al. Circulating concentrations of histamine, neutrophil chemotactic activity, and catecholamines during the refractory period in exercise-induced asthma. J Allergy Clin Immunol 1988;81:100–10.

97. Fish JE, Jameson LS, Albright A, et al. Modulation of the bronchomotor effects of chemical mediators by prostaglandin F alpha in asthmatic subjects. Am Rev Respir Dis 1984;130:571–4.

98. Mattoli S, Foresi A, Corbo GM, et al. The effect of indomethacin on the refractory period occurring after the inhalation of ultrasonically nebulized distilled water. J Allergy Clin Immunol 1987;79:678–83.

99. Margolskee DJ, Bigby BG, Boushey HA. Indomethacin blocks airway tolerance to repetitive exercise but not to eucapnic hyperpnea in asthmatic subjects. Am Rev Respir Dis 1988;137:842–6.

100. O'Byrne PM, Jones GL. The effect of indomethacin on exercise-induced bronchoconstriction and refractoriness after exercise. Am Rev Respir Dis 1986;134:69–72.

101. Manning PJ, Watson RM, O'Byrne PM. Exercise-induced refractoriness in asthmatic subjects involves leukotriene and prostaglandin interdependent mechanisms. Am Rev Respir Dis 1993;148:950–4.

102. Ben-Dov I, Bar-Yishay E, Godfrey S. Refractory period after exercise-induced asthma unexplained by respiratory heat loss. Am Rev Respir Dis 1982;125:530–4.

103. Wilson BA, Bar-Or O, Seed LG. Effects of humid air breathing during arm or treadmill exercise on exercise-induced bronchoconstriction and refractoriness. Am Rev Respir Dis 1990;142:349–52.

104. Wilson BA, Bar-Or O, O'Byrne PM. The effects of indomethacin on refractoriness following exercise both with and without a bronchoconstrictor response. Eur Respir J 1994;7:2174–8.

105. Anderson SD, Daviskas E, Schoeffel RE, et al. Prevention of severe exercise-induced asthma with hot humid air. Lancet 1979;2:629.

106. Hahn AG, Nogrady SG, Burton GR, et al. Absence of refractoriness in asthmatic subjects after exercise with warm, humid inspirate. Allergy Proc 1985;40:418–21.

107. Polosa R. Adenosine-receptor subtypes: their relevance to adenosine-mediated responses in asthma and chronic obstructive pulmonary disease. Eur Respir J 2002;20:488–96.

108. Csoma Z, Huszar E, Vizi E, et al. Adenosine level in exhaled breath increases during exercise-induced bronchoconstriction. Eur Respir J 2005;25:873–8.

109. Magnussen H, Boerger S, Templin K, et al. Effects of a thromboxane-receptor antagonist, BAY u3405, on prostaglandin D and exercise-induced bronchoconstriction. J Allergy Clin Immunol 1992;89:1119–26.

110. Nagakura T, Obata T, Shichijo K, et al. GC/MS analysis of urinary excretion of 9alpha,11beta-PGF2 in acute and exercise-induced asthma in children. Clin Exp Allergy 1998;28:181–6.

111. Anderson SD, Charlton B, Weiler JM, et al. Comparison of mannitol and metha-choline to predict exercise-induced bronchoconstriction and a clinical diagnosis of asthma. Respir Res 2009;23(10):4.
112. Anderson SD, Pearlman DS, Rundell KW, et al. Reproducibility of the airway response to an exercise protocol standardized for intensity, duration, and inspired air conditions, in subjects with symptoms suggestive of asthma. Respir Res 2010;11:120.
113. Mickleborough TD, Lindley MR, Ionescu AA, et al. Protective effect of fish oil supplementation on exercise-induced bronchoconstriction in asthma. Chest 2006;129:39–49.
114. Mickleborough TD, Lindley MR, Ray S. Dietary salt, airway inflammation, and diffusing capacity in exercise-induced asthma. Med Sci Sports Exerc 2005; 37:904–14.
115. Tecklenburg SL, Mickleborough TD, Fly AD, et al. Ascorbic acid supplementation attenuates exercise-induced bronchoconstriction in patients with asthma. Respir Med 2007;101:1770–8.
116. Hemila H. Vitamin C and exercise-induced bronchoconstriction in athletes. J Allergy Clin Immunol 2009;123:274–5.
117. Koh YI, Choi IS. Seasonal difference in the occurrence of exercise-induced bronchospasm In asthmatics: dependence on humidity. Respiration 2002;69: 38–45.
118. Helenius I, Lumme A, Ounap J, et al. No effect of montelukast on asthma-like symptoms in elite ice hockey players. Allergy 2004;59:39–44.
119. Rouhos A, Ekroos H, Karjalainen J, et al. Exhaled nitric oxide and exercise-induced bronchoconstriction in young male conscripts: association only in atopics. Allergy 2005;60:1493–8.
120. Yoshikawa T, Shoji S, Fujii T, et al. Severity of exercise-induced bronchoconstriction is related to airway eosinophilic inflammation in patients with asthma. Eur Respir J 1998;12:879–84.
121. Anderson SD, Holzer K. Exercise-induced asthma: is it the right diagnosis in elite athletes? J Allergy Clin Immunol 2000;106:419–28.
122. Edelman JM, Turpin JA, Bronsky EA, et al. Oral montelukast compared with inhaled salmeterol to prevent exercise-induced bronchoconstriction. A randomized, double-blind trial. Exercise Study Group. Ann Intern Med 2000;132:97–104.
123. Hancox RJ, Subbarao P, Kamada D, et al. Beta2-agonist tolerance and exercise-induced bronchospasm. Am J Respir Crit Care Med 2002;165: 1068–70.
124. Storms W, Chervinsky P, Ghannam AF, et al. A comparison of the effects of oral montelukast and inhaled salmeterol on response to rescue bronchodilation after challenge. Respir Med 2004;98:1051–62.
125. Anderson SD, Caillaud C, Brannan JD. Beta-agonists and exercise-induced asthma. Clin Rev Allergy Immunol 2006;31:163–80.
126. Subbarao P, Duong M, Adelroth E, et al. Effect of ciclesonide dose and duration of therapy on exercise-induced bronchoconstriction in patients with asthma. J Allergy Clin Immunol 2006;117:1008–13.
127. Pearlman DS, van Adelsberg J, Philip G, et al. Onset and duration of protection against exercise-induced bronchoconstriction by a single oral dose of montelukast. Ann Allergy Asthma Immunol 2006;97:98–104.
128. Jonasson G, Carlsen KH, Hultquist C. Low-dose budesonide improves exercise-induced bronchospasm in schoolchildren. Pediatr Allergy Immunol 2000;11: 120–5.

129. Brannan JD, Koskela H, Anderson SD. Monitoring asthma therapy using indirect bronchial provocation tests. Clin Respir J 2007;1:3–15.
130. Knöpfli BH, Bar-Or O. Vagal activity and airway response to ipratropium bromide before and after exercise in ambient and cold conditions in healthy cross-country runners. Clin J Sport Med 1999;9:170–6.
131. Knopfli BH, Bar-Or O, Araujo CG. Effect of ipratropium bromide on EIB in children depends on vagal activity. Med Sci Sports Exerc 2005;37:354–9.
132. van Leeuwen JC, Driessen JM, de Jongh FH, et al. Monitoring pulmonary function during exercise in children with asthma. Arch Dis Child 2011;96:664–8.
133. van Leeuwen JC, Driessen JM, de Jongh FH, et al. Measuring breakthrough exercise-induced bronchoconstriction in young asthmatic children using a jumping castle. J Allergy Clin Immunol 2012. [Epub ahead of print].
134. Vilozni D, Szeinberg A, Barak A, et al. The relation between age and time to maximal bronchoconstriction following exercise in children. Respir Med 2009; 103:1456–60.
135. Hofstra WB, Sterk PJ, Neijens HJ, et al. Prolonged recovery from exercise-induced asthma with increasing age in childhood. Pediatr Pulmonol 1995;20: 177–83.
136. Anderson SD, Lambert S, Brannan JD, et al. Laboratory protocol for exercise asthma to evaluate salbutamol given by two devices. Med Sci Sports Exerc 2001;33:893–900.
137. Schweitzer C, Vu LT, Nguyen YT, et al. Estimation of the bronchodilatory effect of deep inhalation after a free run in children. Eur Respir J 2006;28:89–95.
138. Krishnan R, Trepat X, Nguyen TT, et al. Airway smooth muscle and bronchospasm: fluctuating, fluidizing, freezing. Respir Physiol Neurobiol 2008;163: 17–24.

Index

Note: Page numbers of article titles are in **boldface** type.

Immunol Allergy Clin N Am 33 (2013) 443–448
http://dx.doi.org/10.1016/S0889-8561(13)00048-9
0889-8561/13/$ – see front matter © 2013 Elsevier Inc. All rights reserved.

Printed and bound by CPI Group (UK) Ltd, Croydon, CR0 4YY

03/10/2024

01040489-0017